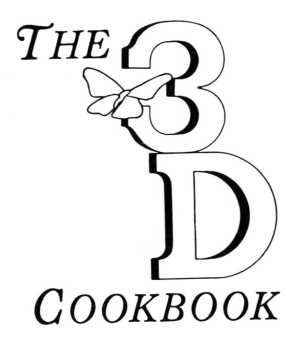

THE 3D COOKBOOK

Paraclete Press
Orleans, Massachusetts

The exchange lists found in the Appendix are based on material in the Exchange Lists for Meal Planning prepared by Committees of the American Diabetes Association, Inc., and the American Dietetic Association, in cooperation with the National Institute of Arthritis, Metabolism and Digestive Diseases and the National Heart and Lung Institute, National Institutes of Health, Public Health Service, U.S. Department of Health, Education and Welfare.

Cover photograph by Everett Sahrbeck
Interior artwork by Doris Carey

First Printing	*July, 1981*
Second Printing	*April, 1982*
Third Printing	*June, 1982*
Fourth Printing	*April, 1983*
Fifth Printing	*January, 1985*
Sixth Printing	*January, 1986*
Seventh Printing	*March, 1987*
Eighth Printing	*March, 1988*

Table of Contents

Soups & Beverages

Breads

Salads

Vegetables

Eggs and Cheese

Chicken

Fish

Meats

8

Desserts

Menu Planning

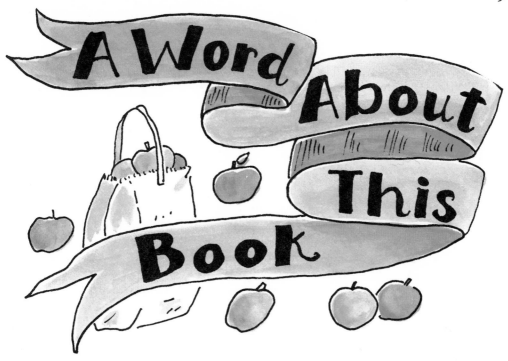

A Word About This Book

Featuring more than 260 delicious, low-calorie recipes, and a time-saving menu-planning section that will be a boon to the harried housewife, this long-awaited cookbook is the answer to a dieter's dream.

In case it may have fallen into the hands of someone who has never heard of 3D, a brief word of explanation seems to be in order. Diet, Discipline & Discipleship — or 3D, for short — is the name of a new Christian diet program that is sweeping the country. It began on Cape Cod, Massachusetts, in 1972, with a group of 40 men and women who wanted help with personal problems in their lives — smoking and drinking, or organizing their time, as well as weight control.

It was agreed that they would meet once a week for eight weeks of facing up to the lack of self-discipline in their lives, in the light of Biblical truth and their Christian commitment. Their pastor turned to the nearby Community of Jesus to provide leadership for the group. Two Community members led the group, and practically everyone benefited a great deal, including a number who had never been able to sustain a diet before, or discover *why* they overate.

Out of this pioneer experience, the program, under the direction of Carol Showalter, who wrote the bestseller *3D*, has grown nationwide, with groups now active in every state and eight foreign countries. Indeed, such has been its remarkable growth that since 1981, more than 80,000 people have participated in 3D, many completing all three of the twelve-week courses offered. (For further information, contact: 3D, P.O. Box 897, Orleans, Massachusetts 02653. 1-800-451-5006).

What's In The Book

The purpose of this book is to make the process of losing weight, if not enjoyable, then at least as painless as possible. It does this primarily through recipes that have been prepared and taste-tested by our 3D staff. These recipes have come to us from 3D-members all over the country, and they provide a stimulating and imaginative combination of taste delights that the whole family will enjoy.

Based on the well-known *Food Exchange Lists*, developed by the American Diabetes Association and the American Dietetic Association, in conjunction with the National Institute for Health, each recipe has the exact exchange equivalents worked out. It is particularly handy, for example, when one is preparing a casserole — for instance Beef-Cabbage Casserole — to know that each portion contains 4 meat exchanges, 2 vegetable exchanges, and ½ fat exchange. The exchanges shown for each recipe will not always appear logical. In calculating them, we worked out the exchange values for each ingredient and fed these into the computer which then gave us the totals of proteins, fats and carbohydrates for the recipe. From these, we worked out the exchanges. It may look like you've lost a half a fat exchange or gained a meat exchange in a given recipe, but stick with it; the final exchanges *are* accurate. For your convenience, the six food exchange lists, and an explanation of how to use them, is contained in the Appendix in the back of this book.

In addition, there is a special section on menu-planning, which will help you to plan meals in advance, using the recipes in this book. The advantages of this are obvious: when you do your shopping, you will be able to confine yourself to only those items which you actually need — thus avoiding "impulse shopping," and often saving considerable time and money, not to mention calories. There are twelve weeks of menus, including many for "special occasions" — those happy, festive times that are like a mine field to the serious dieter.

Best of all, these menus enable the entire family to eat the same thing, while only the dieter (or dieters) will be restricting the quantity of their intake. One of the keys to 3D's phenomenal success is that it re-trains the dieter (and the dieter's family) into well-balanced eating patterns, and the menu planning section will prove most valuable in this regard.

A Word of Thanks

Before we wish you *bon appetit*, we would like to take this opportunity to make special mention of Doris Carey, whose illustrations grace these pages. Also, our thanks go to Loretta Jack, 3D's dietitian, for preparing the diet data in the appendix.

Someday (but not too soon, we hope!) we will be revising this cookbook, and at that time we would very much appreciate any 3D-type recipes that you may have developed on your own, and any comments you may have on the present edition. Please drop us a line at the address mentioned on the preceding page, and may God bless you, as you enjoy this book.

The 3D Staff

From the Director—

It has often been said that 3D is much more than a diet program. Well, the book you hold in your hand is much more than a cookbook — which you have already discovered if you have had a chance to read the preceding note about what's in it, and how to use it.

We would like to draw your attention here to the personal element that has gone into its preparation. One of the things that happens in a 3D group during the course of a twelve-week session is that the members are drawn very close — not just through the shared mutual needs and the daily praying for one another, but through experiencing God's encouragement and healing touch operating through the group.

When the group completes a session, there is often a desire to carry on in some way, and many continue on to a second or third session. A sense of family has developed among the members, and in a surprising way this seems to extend to include all those involved in 3D groups, past and present. Long before we came to see how useful a 3D cookbook might be, 3D-ers began sending in recipes — either for our newsletter, 3D Living Free, or simply for the folks in the home office to enjoy.

When the cookbook project was actually begun, it, too, was a family affair. Anyone who wanted to work on it was welcome; we needed all the help we could get. Anyway, we hope that some of the family feeling has gotten through to the pages and that this book will be a blessing.

Bon Appetit!

Carol Showalter

Carol Showalter

Ho, every one who thirsts, come to the waters; and he who has no money, come, buy wine and milk without money and without price.

Isaiah 55:1

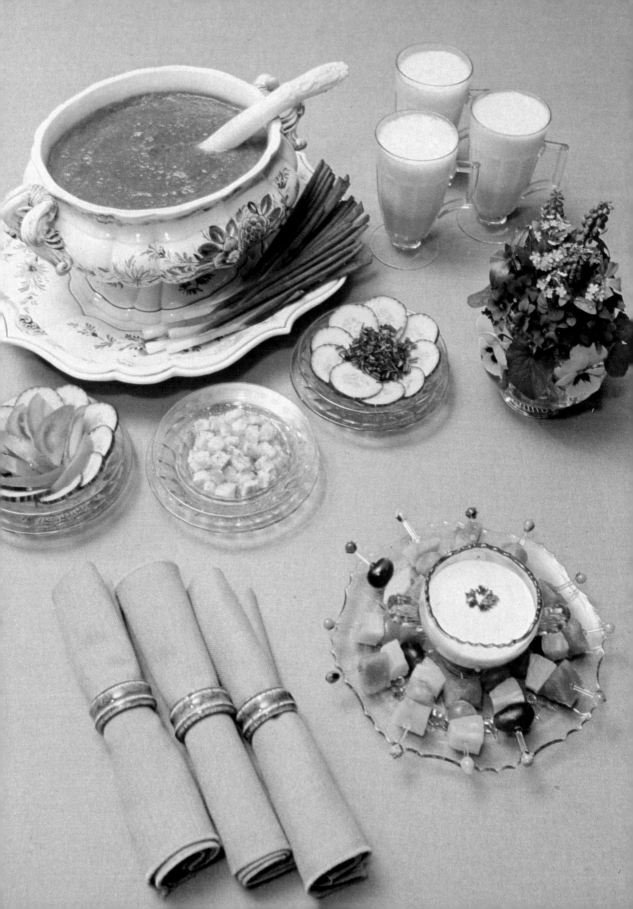

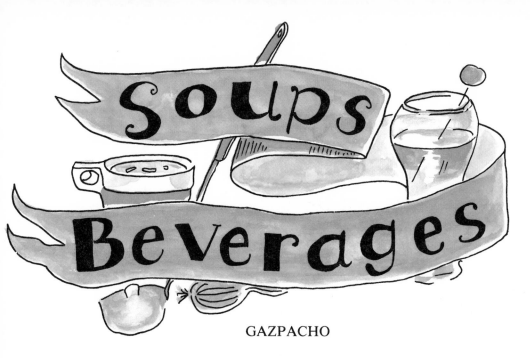

GAZPACHO

3 large tomatoes, peeled, seeded and chopped
  fine
3 green onions with tops, sliced thin
1 large green pepper, seeded and chopped
1 medium cucumber, peeled, seeded and
  chopped
3 tablespoons minced parsley
1 large clove garlic, crushed
1 (10¾-ounce) can condensed chicken broth
1 soup can water
¼ cup red wine vinegar
2 tablespoons olive oil
salt and pepper to taste
½ cup coarse bread crumbs

In large bowl mix well tomatoes, onions,
  green pepper, cucumber, parsley, garlic,
  broth, water, vinegar and oil.
Add salt and pepper.
Cover and chill 2 hours to allow flavors to
  blend.
To serve, sprinkle with crumbs.
Serves 5   each: 1 Bread Exchange
                      1 Vegetable Exchange
                      1 Fat Exchange

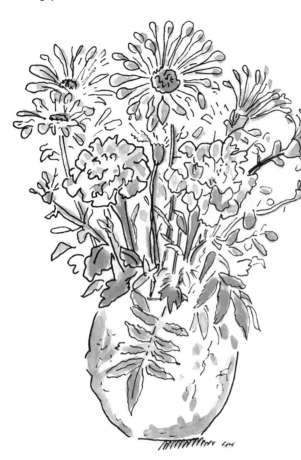

EASY VEGETABLE SOUP

1 ½ pounds lean ground beef
½ cup chopped onions
½ cup diced potatoes
½ cup sliced carrots
¼ cup chopped celery
½ cup shredded cabbage
1 cup canned tomatoes
3 cups water
⅛ cup rice
½ bay leaf
¼ teaspoon thyme
½ basil leaf
2 teaspoons salt
⅛ teaspoon pepper
¼ cup grated cheddar cheese

Cook ground beef and onions in skillet until
    meat is brown; carefully drain meat and
    blot with paper towels to remove all grease.
Combine meat and all remaining ingredients
    in large skillet.
Simmer until vegetables are tender.

Serves 6   each: 2 Meat Exchanges
                                   1 Bread Exchange
                                   2 Vegetable Exchanges
                                   2 Fat Exchanges

LIFE SAVER SOUP

½ head cabbage, shredded
1 large can of tomatoes
4 stalks of celery, diced
4 tablespoons onion flakes
4 beef bouillon cubes
3 quarts water
1 teaspoon oregano
1 tablespoon parsley flakes

Combine all ingredients together and simmer
    3 hours.

Serves 6   each: 2 Vegetable Exchanges

MEATBALL SOUP

4 cups beef broth
1 pound extra lean ground beef
1 egg
½ teaspoon salt
¼ teaspoon pepper
10 green onions with tops, cut in ½-inch pieces
1 cup thinly sliced celery
1 cup thinly sliced carrots
2 tomatoes, peeled and cut in eighths
½ cup rice
1 bay leaf
1 teaspoon basil
2-3 tablespoons soy sauce
2 tablespoons minced parsley

In large pot, heat broth to simmer.
Mix beef, egg, salt and pepper; shape in 1½-inch balls.
Brown meatballs and drain off all fat.
Drop into broth.
Add onions, celery, carrots, tomatoes, rice, bay leaf and basil.
Cover and simmer 35 minutes, stirring occasionally.
Discard bay leaf.
Stir in soy sauce.
Top each serving with parsley.
Serves 6   each: 2 Meat Exchanges
                        1 Bread Exchange
                        1 Vegetable Exchange

VEGETABLE SOUP

2 medium carrots
6 stalks celery
1 medium Bermuda onion
¼ cup safflower oil
8 ounces tomato juice
5 ripe tomatoes, blended
2 cups vegetable cooking water
1 small zucchini, chopped
1 cup cooked brown rice or garbanzos
½ cup shredded cabbage
3 tablespoons soy sauce
Assorted herbs to taste
1½ cups cottage cheese

Chop carrot, celery, onion.
Saute in oil about 10 minutes.
Add tomato juice, blended tomatoes, and vegetable cooking water.
Add zucchini, cooked rice or garbanzos, cabbage, soy sauce and assorted herbs to tomato broth.
Cook until tender, about 5-10 minutes.
Vegetables should be firm.
Add ¼ cup of cottage cheese to each bowl of soup.
Serves 6   each: 1 Meat Exchange
                        1 Bread Exchange
                        2 Vegetable Exchanges
                        2 Fat Exchanges

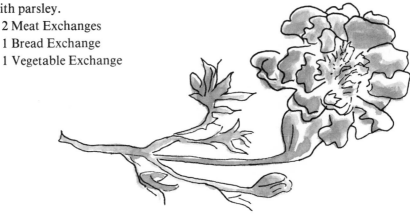

CREAM OF CELERY SOUP

2 stalks of celery (diced small)
½ cup mushrooms (optional)
2 teaspoons chopped onion
1 bouillon cube — chicken or beef
dash of garlic powder or your favorite spice
1 cup skim milk
1 teaspoon cornstarch

Bring to a boil the first 5 ingredients in ½ cup
  water and simmer 20-30 minutes.
Add milk mixed with cornstarch.
Bring to a boil and simmer 2-3 minutes.
Serves 2   each: 1 Vegetable Exchange
                       ½ Milk Exchange

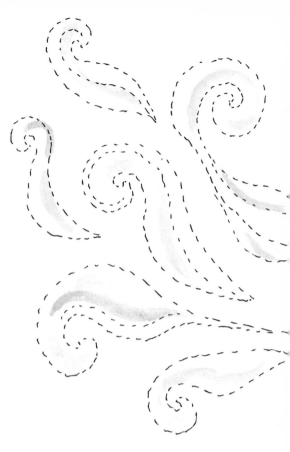

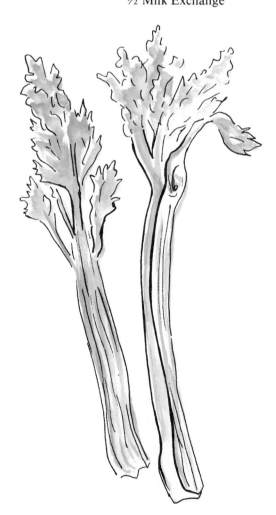

ZESTY TOMATO CABBAGE SOUP

1 (46-ounce) can V-8 juice
2 beef-flavor bouillon cubes or envelopes
1 medium head cabbage, coarsely shredded
1 cup water
1 medium onion, sliced
1 garlic clove, minced
1 tablespoon salt
1 tablespoon sugar
1 tablespoon lemon juice
¼ teaspoon hot pepper sauce

Combine all ingredients in a 4-quart saucepan; cook over medium-high heat until
  boiling.
Reduce heat to low, cover and simmer 30
  minutes or until cabbage is tender.
Serves 10   each: 1 Vegetable Exchange

ASPARAGUS SOUP

1 small can asparagus, undrained
1 (16-ounce) can green beans, undrained
1 beef bouillon cube

Place all ingredients in blender.
Blend until consistency of soup.

Serves 4   each: 2 Vegetable Exchanges

CREAM OF TOMATO SOUP

1 (18-ounce) can tomato juice
½ teaspoon instant minced onion
2-3 dashes Worcestershire sauce
6 tablespoons skim milk powder
Salt as desired

Mix ingredients together and simmer for a few minutes.

Serves 3   each: 1 Vegetable Exchange
                     ½ Milk Exchange

VEGETABLE CHEESE SOUP/SAUCE

½ cup chopped celery
½ cup green pepper
½ cup scallions or onions
1 tablespoon butter
2 tablespoons flour
1½ cups skim milk
4 ounces diet cheese
1 cup chicken broth or bouillon (for sauce, eliminate broth)

In large skillet saute celery, peppers and
   onions in butter for 5 minutes.
Do not overcook.
Salt and pepper to taste.
Shake flour with ½ cup milk, mix well, add
   to vegetables with remaining cup of milk.
Simmer slowly, stirring until thickened.
Add cheese and chicken broth.
When using as a sauce, serve over boiled or
   broiled fish.

Serves 4   each: 1 Meat Exchange
                     1 Milk Exchange
                     1 Fat Exchange

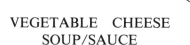
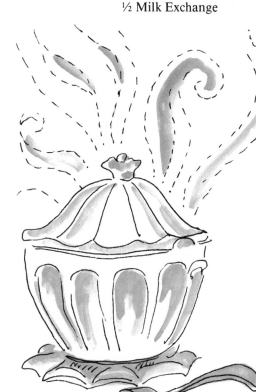

CABBAGE SOUP

1 onion, sliced thin
1 medium tomato, peeled and chopped
1 carrot, shredded
¼ cup celery, chopped
1 bay leaf
¼ teaspoon caraway seeds
white pepper
salt
½ clove garlic, minced or crushed
2 cups green cabbage, shredded or sliced
  paper-thin
1 can consomme
yogurt

Put all the ingredients except cabbage and
  consomme in a pan.
Add enough water to cover.
Bring to a boil and cook 15 minutes.
Add cabbage and cook 10 more minutes.
Serve topped with 1 tablespoon yogurt.
Serves 4   each: 1 Vegetable Exchange

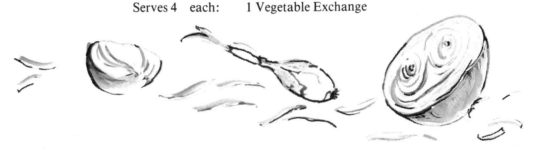

FRENCH ONION SOUP I

1½ pounds onions, thinly sliced
2 tablespoons butter
4 cups prepared beef bouillon
1 teaspoon Worcestershire sauce
6 slices French bread, toasted
grated Parmesan cheese

In covered pan, cook onions in butter until
  tender.
Add beef bouillon, Worcestershire sauce and
  a dash of pepper.
Bring to a boil.
Sprinkle toast slices with cheese; place under
  broiler until cheese is lightly browned.
Ladle soup into bowls and float toast on top.

Serves 6   each: 1 Bread Exchange
                    2 Vegetable Exchanges
                    1 Fat Exchange

JUNE'S SOUP

1 head of cabbage
2 large onions
1 large bunch celery
1 large green pepper
1 can whole tomatoes
2 packages onion soup mix

Cut vegetables in bite-size pieces and cover
  with water.
Simmer until vegetables are tender, and add
  onion soup mix.
Parmesan cheese may be sprinkled over each
  bowl of soup.
Serves 12   each: 1 Vegetable Exchange
                       ½ Bread Exchange

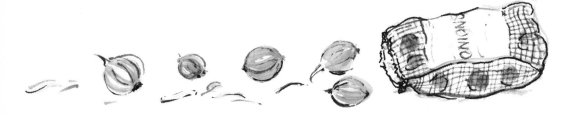

FRENCH ONION SOUP II

5 cups strong beef bouillon
6 large onions, thinly sliced
4 tablespoons margarine
Salt and pepper
½ teaspoon ground thyme
1 teaspoon paprika
2 cloves garlic, crushed
1 bayleaf
Croutons
1 cup grated Swiss and Parmesan cheese
  mixed together

Heat margarine in a large saucepan.
Add onions and fry quickly until evenly
  cooked.
Add seasonings, bouillon and simmer one
  hour.
At serving time heat to rolling boil and ladle
  into serving bowls.
Cover with croutons and cheese and place
  under broiler until cheese melts.
Serve immediately.

Serves 6 each (without cheese and croutons):
                1 Vegetable Exchange
                2 Fat Exchanges
½ cup croutons = 1 Bread Exchange
1 ounce cheese = 1 Meat Exchange

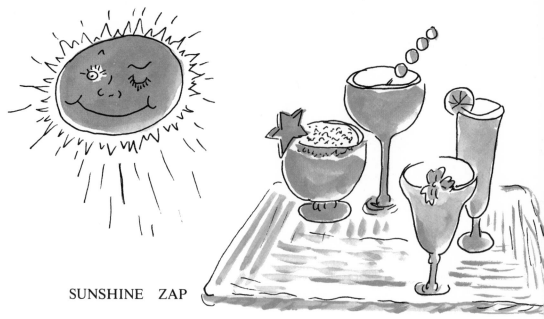

SUNSHINE ZAP

2 cups unsweetened orange juice
*1½ medium-size bananas (approximately 1
   cup)*
1 cup unsweetened pineapple juice
3 ice cubes

Put all ingredients except ice cubes into
   blender and process until fruit is liquefied.
Add ice cubes and blend a few seconds longer.
Serve immediately.
Serves 8   each: 1 Fruit Exchange

AMBROSIA   SHAKE

4 ripe bananas
⅓ cup orange juice
¼ teaspoon almond extract
1 quart cold skim milk

Blend bananas, orange juice and almond
   extract in blender.
Add milk and beat well.
Serves 6   each: 1 Fruit Exchange
                      1 Milk Exchange

MINT   BERRY   SPLASH

6 tablespoons instant tea powder
½ cup sugar or sweetener to equal ½ cup
2 quarts water
1 quart cranberry juice
1 cup orange juice
⅔ cup lemon juice
½ teaspoon cinnamon
¼ teaspoon nutmeg
Fresh mint

Combine all ingredients and stir.
Garnish with mint leaves or orange slices.
Makes 1 gallon.
Serves 32   each: 1 Fruit Exchange
                       (1 cup serving if using
sweetener, ½ cup serving if using sugar)

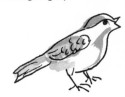

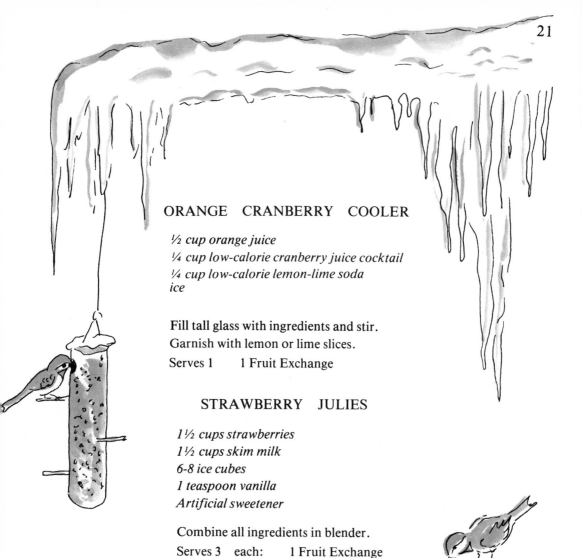

ORANGE CRANBERRY COOLER

½ cup orange juice
¼ cup low-calorie cranberry juice cocktail
¼ cup low-calorie lemon-lime soda
ice

Fill tall glass with ingredients and stir.
Garnish with lemon or lime slices.
Serves 1   1 Fruit Exchange

STRAWBERRY JULIES

1½ cups strawberries
1½ cups skim milk
6-8 ice cubes
1 teaspoon vanilla
Artificial sweetener

Combine all ingredients in blender.
Serves 3   each: 1 Fruit Exchange
                         ½ Milk Exchange

BERRY SHAKE

1 cup skim milk
½ cup frozen berries
Artificial sweetener to taste
2 ice cubes

Combine all ingredients in blender.
Blend at highest speed for 30 seconds.
Substitute vanilla, rum or peppermint extract
    for fruit if you do not wish to use your fruit
    allowance.
Serves 1   1 Fruit Exchange
                1 Milk Exchange

STRAWBERRY SODA

1 cup strawberries
1 cup skim milk
Artificial sweetener (optional)
Low-calorie ginger ale

Blend strawberries and milk in blender at
    medium speed.
Sweeten with sweetener if desired.
Add ginger ale for an ice cream soda effect.
Serves 2   each: ½ Fruit Exchange
                         ½ Milk Exchange

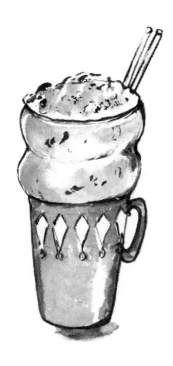

PINK   LEMONADE

1 cup fresh lemon juice
2 cups unsweetened red grape juice, undiluted
Artificial sweetener to taste

Combine ingredients in a small covered jar
   and shake well.
Store in the refrigerator and shake before
   using.
To make a glass of lemonade, combine ⅓ cup
   with cold water and ice cubes in a tall glass.
Serves 9   each: 1 Fruit Exchange

CANTALOUPE   MILKSHAKE

½ cantaloupe
⅔ cup low-calorie lemon-lime soda
⅓ cup dry milk
1 teaspoon vanilla
8-10 ice cubes
Artificial sweetener to taste

Combine all ingredients in blender.
Blend at medium-high speed; add ice cubes
   one at a time.
Serve immediately.
Serves 2   each: 1 Fruit Exchange
                              ½ Milk Exchange

BANANA   MILKSHAKE

1 cup skim milk
1 ripe banana
3 ice cubes

Put in blender on highest speed
   for 30 seconds.
Serves 1   2 Fruit Exchanges
                    1 Milk Exchange

ORANGE MILKSHAKE

1 cup orange juice
⅓ cup skim milk powder
2 eggs
1 teaspoon vanilla
dash of salt
nutmeg, if desired

Blend all ingredients in a blender, adding
   each one at a time.

   Serves 2   each: 1 Meat Exchange
                        1 Fruit Exchange
                        ½ Milk Exchange
                        1 Fat Exchange

PINEAPPLE SLUSH

2 cups diced fresh pineapple or canned in its
   own juice, drained
2 cups crushed ice
6 whole strawberries

In a blender, blend pineapple and ice 10
   seconds at low speed.
Pour into glasses.
Garnish with strawberries.
Serves 6   each: 1 Fruit Exchange

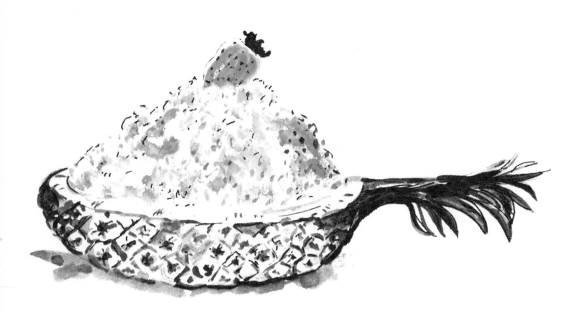

Jesus said to them, "I am the bread of life. He who comes to me shall never hunger, and he who believes in me shall never thirst."

John 6:35

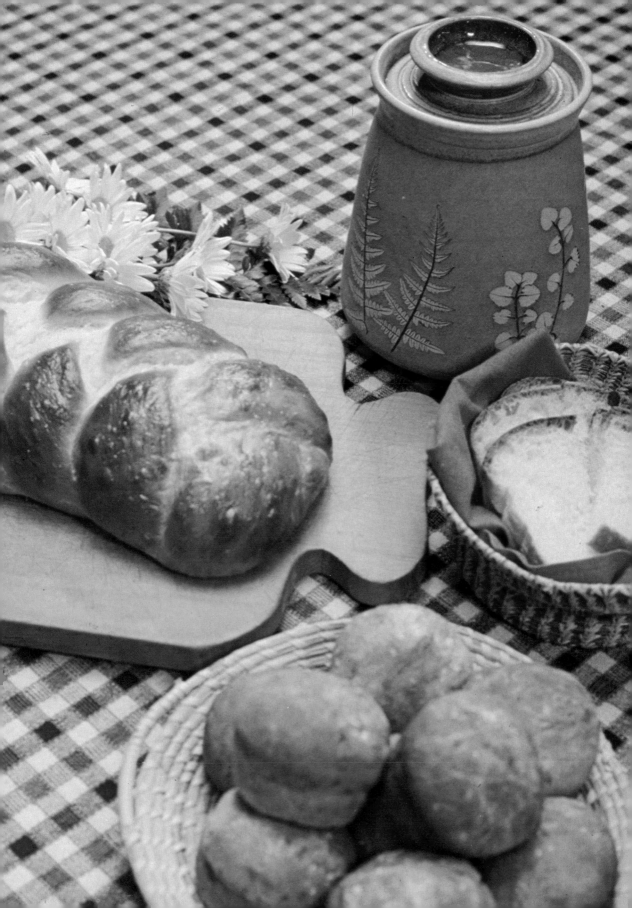

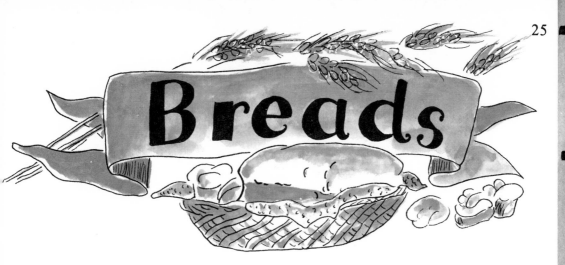

Breads

RYE ROLLS

1 yeast cake or 1 package dry yeast
¼ cup warm water
1 cup small curd cottage cheese
2 tablespoons sugar
¼ teaspoon baking soda
1 egg, lightly beaten
2 tablespoons caraway seeds
1 teaspoon salt
1 cup all-purpose flour
1 cup rye flour

Soften yeast in ¼ cup warm water.
Warm cottage cheese in saucepan.
Add yeast in water to the warm cottage cheese.
Add sugar, soda, beaten egg, caraway seeds and salt.
Mix well.
Add the flour a little at a time, mixing well.
Cover and allow to stand at room temperature for several hours or until doubled in bulk.
Stir dough until reduced to original size.
Shape into rolls and put in well-greased flat 9x13'' pan.
Cover and again allow dough to double in bulk.
Bake at 350° for 30-40 minutes.
Serves 12   each: 1½ Bread Exchanges

POTATO BREAD

1 package yeast
3½ cups flour
¼ cup sugar
1½ teaspoons salt
1 cup mashed potato — unseasoned
⅔ cup milk
¼ cup melted margarine
2 eggs

Mix yeast, 1½ cups flour, sugar and salt.
Heat milk and butter. Cool until lukewarm.
  Stir into flour mixture with potato and eggs.
Beat 2 minutes.
Stir in 1 cup flour and then remaining flour
  until easy to handle.
Knead 8-10 minutes.
Place in greased bowl, turn greased side up,
  cover and let rise until double, 1½-2 hours.
Punch down and divide into thirds.
Roll into rope 14 inches long.
Braid on greased cookie sheet.
Don't stretch dough.
Tuck ends under.
Let rise 45 minutes.
Brush top with egg white and 1 teaspoon
  of water.
May put sesame or poppy seeds on top.
Bake at 350° for 30-35 minutes.

30 slices   each: 1 Bread Exchange
                    ½ Fat Exchange

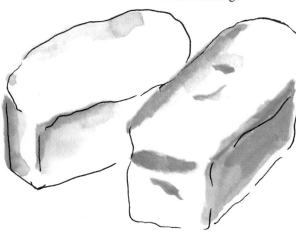

WHEAT-GERM ROLLS

1 cup warm milk
¼ cup honey
2 packages dry yeast
⅓ cup oil
1 egg
½ cup wheat germ
2 teaspoons salt
2½ cups whole wheat flour

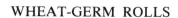

Combine milk, honey and yeast and let set 5
  minutes.
Add rest of ingredients.
Mix well and knead. Let rise in warm place
  until double.
Punch down and form into rolls. Let rise
  again. Bake in preheated oven at 375° for
  20-25 minutes.

Serves 12   each: 2 Bread Exchanges
                    1½ Fat Exchanges

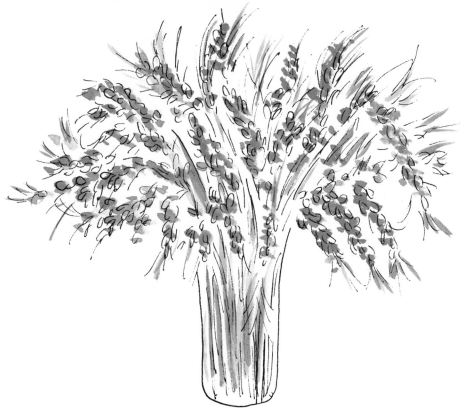

JUANITA'S WHEAT MUFFINS

¾ cup unbleached white flour
1 teaspoon salt
1 teaspoon baking soda
1 teaspoon baking powder
1½ cups whole wheat flour
1 egg
½ cup vegetable oil
½ cup honey
1 cup buttermilk or sour milk

Sift white flour, salt, baking soda and baking powder into medium-size bowl.

Stir in wheat flour.

Combine oil, honey, buttermilk and egg in small bowl; pour into dry ingredients.

Mix just until dry ingredients are moistened.

Fill well-greased 2½-inch muffin cups ⅔ full.

Bake at 400° for 15 minutes.

Remove to wire racks.

Serve warm.

Serves 18   each: 1½ Bread Exchanges
1 Fat Exchange

BROWN GRAHAM BREAD

2 cups wheat flour
1 cup white flour
½ cup corn meal
¼ cup sugar
2 teaspoons baking soda
1 teaspoon baking powder
1 teaspoon salt
½ cup molasses
2 cups sour milk
1 cup raisins
nutmeg as desired

Mix all dry ingredients together in large bowl.

Blend in molasses and sour milk.

Fold in raisins.

Pour batter into 2 small loaf pans, well greased.

Bake at 350° for 35-40 minutes.

Each loaf makes 15 slices.

1 slice = 1 Bread Exchange

bread

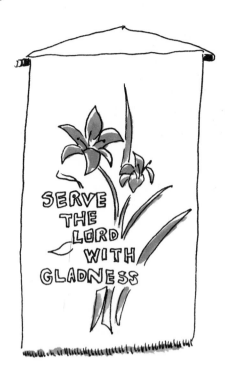

SERVE THE LORD WITH GLADNESS

BAKED FRENCH TOAST

1 medium egg
1 teaspoon water
dash of salt
dash of vanilla
1 slice raisin bread

In shallow bowl combine egg, water, salt
  and vanilla.
Soak bread in mixture until all liquid is absorbed, turning at least once.
Place bread on non-stick baking sheet and
  bake at 350° for 10-12 minutes or until
  lightly browned.
Spread with 1 teaspoon butter.
Serves 1   1 Meat Exchange
                        1 Bread Exchange
                        1 Fat Exchange

ORANGE FRENCH TOAST

6 eggs
1 cup orange juice
1 teaspoon sugar
¼ teaspoon salt
12 slices French bread
2 tablespoons butter or margarine

Beat together eggs, orange juice, sugar and
  salt.
Dip bread into egg mixture, coating both
  sides.
Place bread on non-stick shallow baking
  pan.
Melt butter; drizzle over bread.
Bake at 500° for 5 minutes.
Turn and bake until golden, about 5 minutes
  more.
Serves 6   each: 1 Meat Exchange
                    2 Bread Exchanges
                    2 Fat Exchanges
Serve with Orange Sauce, page 155.

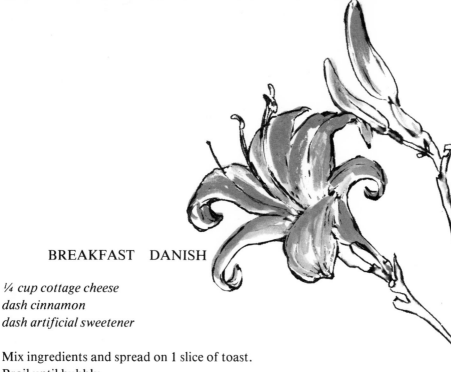

BREAKFAST DANISH

¼ cup cottage cheese
dash cinnamon
dash artificial sweetener

Mix ingredients and spread on 1 slice of toast.
Broil until bubbly.
Serves 1   1 Bread Exchange
                 1 Meat Exchange

OVERNIGHT FRENCH TOAST

4 eggs
½ cup skim milk
2 teaspoons honey
dash of cinnamon

Place 6 slices day old, whole wheat bread
    in 9x13-inch pan.
Pour egg mixture over bread, moving and
    turning it so that all bread is completely
    covered.
Cover and store overnight in refrigerator.
Next morning, remove bread with spatula
    and fry on lightly buttered hot griddle until
    golden brown, turning once only.
Serve with sliced fruit or berries or hot apple
    sauce.
Serves 6   each: 1 Meat Exchange
                        1 Bread Exchange

bread

BREAKFAST COBBLER

1 egg
½ cup skim milk
1 diced apple
1 slice of bread
½ teaspoon vanilla
⅛ teaspoon cinnamon
⅛ teaspoon butter
¼ teaspoon almond flavoring
sweetener to taste

Beat egg.
Add skim milk, crumbled bread, diced apple
   and flavoring.
Put in small baking dish.
Bake 20 minutes at 350°.
Sprinkle sweetener on top.
Serves 1   1 Meat Exchange
                   1 Bread Exchange
                   1 Fruit Exchange
                   ½ Milk Exchange
                   1 Fat Exchange

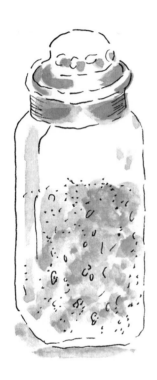

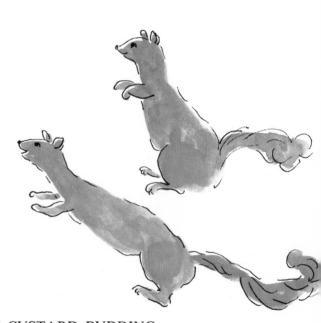

BREAKFAST CUSTARD PUDDING

1 cup skim milk
1 medium egg, beaten
1 slice white bread, crumbled
½ teaspoon vanilla extract
½ teaspoon cinnamon
½ teaspoon nutmeg
sweetener to taste

Combine all ingredients in a medium bowl.
Pour into 10-ounce custard cup.
Bake at 350° 20-25 minutes or until top is
   puffed and lightly browned.
Serves 1   1 Meat Exchange
                   1 Bread Exchange
                   1 Milk Exchange
                   ½ Fat Exchange

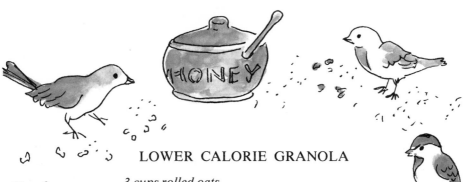

LOWER CALORIE GRANOLA

3 cups rolled oats
1½ cups wheat germ
¼ cup dry milk
¼ cup chopped nuts or seeds
½ cup raisins
⅓ cup oil
⅓ cup honey
¼ teaspoon cinnamon
1 teaspoon vanilla extract

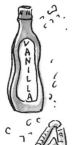
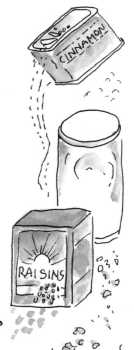
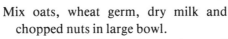
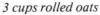

Mix oats, wheat germ, dry milk and chopped nuts in large bowl.

Heat and stir oil and honey in small saucepan until blended (about 2 minutes).

Remove from heat and stir in cinnamon and vanilla.

Drizzle honey mixture over oat mixture and stir thoroughly.

Spread on 2 cookie sheets and bake at 300° for 10 minutes.

Remove and stir well.

Bake 10 minutes more, remove and stir.

Bake 5 minutes more.

Cool completely; add raisins and store in airtight container.

Serve with skim milk.

Serves 24   each: 1 bread Exchange
1 Fruit Exchange
1 Fat Exchange

Each serving ¼ cup.

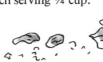

bread

APPLE WHOLE WHEAT PANCAKES

2 cups whole wheat flour
2 eggs
2 cups skim milk
2 medium cooking apples
1 teaspoon cinnamon
2 tablespoons vegetable oil
1 tablespoon honey
2 teaspoons baking powder
½ teaspoon salt
½ teaspoon nutmeg

Grate apple (approximately 1 cup).
Beat eggs and combine apple, milk, honey and oil.
Mix together flour, salt, baking powder and spices.
Add liquid ingredients and stir.
Cook pancakes on lightly oiled hot griddle.

Serves 6   each: 2 Bread Exchanges
                                  1 Milk Exchange
                                  1 Fat Exchange

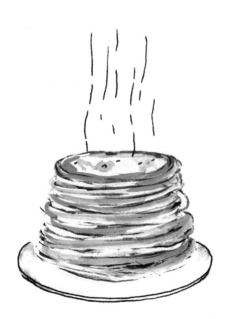

BACON & CHEESE OVEN PANCAKES

6 slices bacon
1 cup flour
1½ tablespoons sugar
1 tablespoon baking powder
½ teaspoon salt
1 egg, beaten
¾ cup skim milk
1 cup shredded sharp cheese

Cook bacon until crisp; drain well on paper towels.
Crumble and set aside.
Reserve 1 tablespoon of drippings.
In bowl stir together flour, sugar, baking powder and salt.

Combine eggs, milk and reserved drippings.
Add all at once to dry ingredients, beating until smooth.
Stir in bacon.
Spray baking pan (15x10x1-inch) with non-stick spray.
Spread batter evenly in pan.
Bake 425° oven for 15 minutes.
Sprinkle with cheese, bake 2-3 minutes more till cheese is melted.

Serves 6   each: 1 Meat Exchange
                                  1 Bread Exchange
                                  2 Fat Exchanges

BLUEBERRY PANCAKES

1½ cups flour
½ teaspoon baking soda
1 teaspoon salt
½ teaspoon nutmeg
1 egg, beaten
8 ounces plain yogurt
1 cup skim milk
1 cup unsweetened fresh or frozen blueberries

Stir dry ingredients together.
Beat egg, yogurt and milk until smooth.
Add to dry ingredients and stir to combine.
Fold in blueberries.
Drop ¼ cup for each pancake on non-stick
　griddle.
Serve with Hot Blueberry Syrup:

1 cup unsweetened blueberries
½ cup unsweetened grape juice

Combine in saucepan and bring to boil.
Crush berries with spoon and simmer 2-3
　minutes.
Serve hot.
Serves 8　each with Hot Blueberry Syrup
　　　　　　　　¼ Meat Exchange
　　　　　　　　1 Bread Exchange
　　　　　　　　1 Fruit Exchange

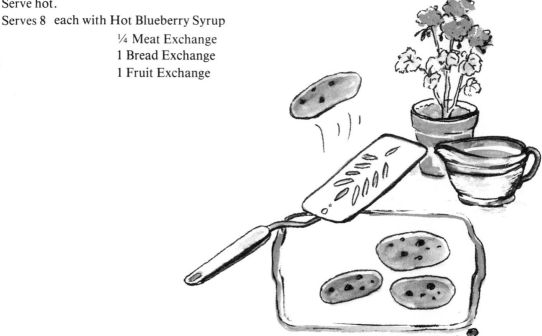

bread

BRAN MUFFINS

1½ cups whole wheat flour
3 teaspoons baking powder
1 teaspoon salt
⅓ cup honey
1½ cups Kellogg's Bran Buds
⅓ cup vegetable oil
1 cup skim milk
1 egg
½ cup raisins

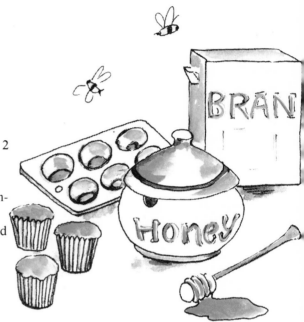

Combine flour, baking powder, salt.
Add Bran Buds to milk and let set for 2 minutes.
Add eggs, oil and honey to bran mixture.
Stir in dry ingredients, mixing only until combined.
Bake at 400° 20-25 minutes in paper-lined muffin cups.
Serves 24, each muffin 1 Bread Exchange
                    1 Fat Exchange

WORKING WOMAN'S
BRAN MUFFINS

2 cups boiling water
2 cups Kellogg's Bran buds
1 cup shortening (heaping)
4 eggs
1 quart buttermilk
5 cups flour
5 teaspoons baking soda
1 teaspoon salt
4 cups Kellogg's All Bran
1 cup raisins

Combine boiling water and Bran Buds and let stand.
Combine shortening and eggs, adding 1 egg at a time and beating well.

Add the remaining 5 ingredients.
Now add the Bran Bud mixture that you had let stand.
Add the raisins.
Store in container in refrigerator (covered).
Do not stir again when taking out of container.
Use ¼ cup batter for each muffin.
Bake at 400° 20-25 minutes in paper-lined muffin cups.
Makes 64 muffins, each: 1 Bread Exchange
                          1 Fat Exchange

Keeps 7 weeks.

JOHNNY CAKE (CORNBREAD)

1 cup flour
1 cup cornmeal
1 cup milk
½ cup sugar
1 egg, well beaten
pinch of salt
½ teaspoon soda
1 teaspoon cream of tartar
1 tablespoon molasses
1 tablespoon butter, melted

Sift dry ingredients together in a bowl.
Add other ingredients and beat thoroughly.
Pour into shallow greased baking pan and
  bake in a hot (375°) oven for 30 minutes.
Serves 15   each: 1 Bread Exchange

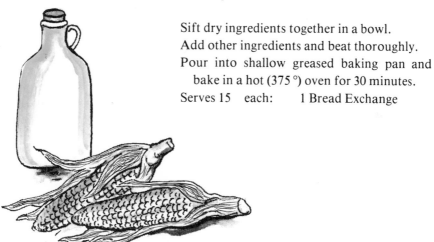

CRANBERRY BREAD

2 eggs
¼ cup water
12 slices dry bread, rolled into crumbs
⅔ cup dry milk powder
1 teaspoon grated orange rind
1 teaspoon vanilla extract
¼ teaspoon baking soda
2 cups fresh or frozen cranberries
  (no sugar added)
Artificial sweetener to equal 6 teaspoons
  sugar

Combine all ingredients except cranberries in
  blender.
Whip for 1 minute ; add to cranberries in
  bowl.
Mix well; pour into 10-inch teflon pan and
  bake at 350° for 35-40 minutes until top is
  puffed and lightly brown.
Serves 9   each slice: 1 Bread Exchange

bread

POTATOES AU GRATIN

3 potatoes, peeled, boiled and sliced
½ cup celery chunks
1 (10¾-ounce) can cheddar cheese soup
1 tablespoon prepared mustard

Arrange the potato slices and the celery chunks in a non-stick baking dish.
Mix the cheese soup and the mustard together in a bowl, and pour this mixture over the potatoes.
Bake at 375° for 30 minutes.
Serves 8   each: 1 Bread Exchange
                              1 Fat Exchange

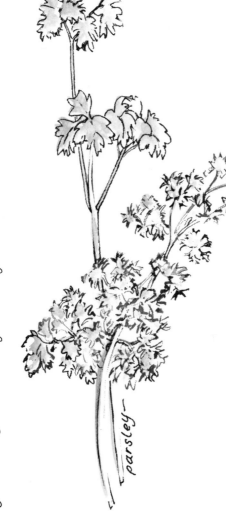

always have parsley on hand to use as a garnish ~ or to snip and add for its flavor.

parsley

STUFFED IDAHO POTATOES

6 medium Idaho potatoes
¾ cup hot skim milk
1 teaspoon minced onion
1 teaspoon salt, dash of pepper
1 egg separated
2 tablespoons grated American cheese

Scrub potatoes, pierce and bake until tender.
Cut a slice from the top of the potato and scoop out the solids.
Use the solids from 3 potatoes, reserving the rest for another meal.
Add milk, onion, salt, pepper and egg yolk.
Mix with electric mixer until creamy.
Beat egg white until stiff; set aside.
Fold beaten egg white into mixture.
Fill potato shells and sprinkle with grated cheese.
Bake at 350° for 20 minutes or until heated through.
The mixture thickens as it heats.
Serves 6   each: ½ Meat Exchange
                              1 Bread Exchange

RICE AND MUSHROOMS

1 (10½-ounce) can condensed beef or chicken
   broth
1 (4-ounce) can sliced mushrooms, drained,
   reserving liquid
2 medium onions, chopped
½ cup wild rice
1 cup long grain rice
2 tablespoons parsley

Skim any visible fat from broth.
Add water to broth to make 2 cups.
Boil broth, mushroom liquid and onions in a
   saucepan.
Add wild rice, reduce heat and simmer
   20 minutes.
Add regular rice and mushrooms.
Boil again and simmer 20 minutes until ten-
   der.
Garnish with parsley.
Serves 10   each: 1 Bread Exchange
                       1 Vegetable Exchange

HERBED SAFFRON RICE

1½ pounds converted rice
¼ cup butter
1 package saffron threads
2 quarts chicken broth
1 teaspoon crumbled basil
1 tablespoon dillweed
1¼ cups sliced scallions
salt and pepper

In a 2½- to 3-quart saucepan, mix the rice
   and butter and stir over a moderate heat
   until the rice is lightly browned.
Stir in saffron, chicken broth, basil and dill.
Simmer, stirring occasionally, until the rice is
   tender and the liquid is absorbed.
Season with salt and pepper and stir in the
   scallions.
Serves 8   each: 2 Bread Exchanges
                       1 Fat Exchange

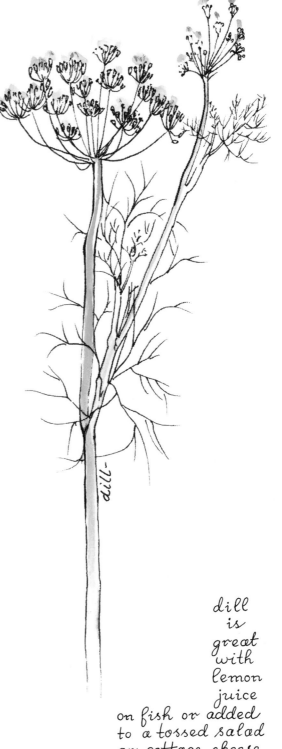

dill

bread

dill is great with lemon juice on fish or added to a tossed salad or cottage cheese

CORNBREAD STUFFING

1 small onion, chopped
1 sweet pepper, minced
2 stalks celery, diced
1 cup chicken bouillon or clear broth
1 small package seasoned cornbread mix
1 egg

Spray teflon skillet with non-stick spray.
Saute onion, pepper and celery until tender.
Add bouillon or broth.
Simmer for 2-3 minutes.
To cornbread mix, add egg and vegetables in broth.
Bake at 325° approximately 45 minutes.
Add more or less broth for dry or moist dressing as you prefer.
Variations on Dressing:
Substitute 1 cup cooked rice for cornbread mix or
1 cup cooked eggplant for cornbread mix.

Serves 8   each: 1 Bread Exchange
1 Vegetable Exchange
1 Fat Exchange

APPLE-BACON POULTRY STUFFING

6 apples, peeled and chopped
2 cups cubed bread, lightly toasted
½ cup chopped onion
½ cup cubed Canadian bacon
1 cup minced celery
¼ cup chopped parsley
1 teaspoon salt
¼ teaspoon pepper
1 teaspoon poultry seasoning
½ cup hot giblet stock or boiling water

Combine all the ingredients, mixing them lightly.
Loosely fill the cavity of a turkey, chicken or rock Cornish hen.
The stuffing can also be baked in a 1½-quart casserole in a preheated 350° oven for 45 minutes.

Serves 6   each: 1 Bread Exchange
1 Vegetable Exchange
1 Fruit Exchange
1 Fat Exchange

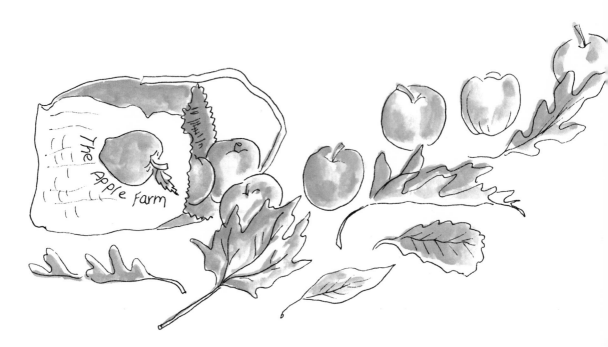

PEAS WITH MUSHROOMS

1 pound shelled peas (3 cups)
¾ cup canned or fresh mushrooms
1 small onion, sliced in circles
1 teaspoon butter
Salt and pepper to taste

Cook peas and onion circles until tender (about 15 minutes).
Meanwhile, brown mushrooms in butter.
Combine.
Add salt and pepper to taste.

Serves 6   each: ½ Bread Exchange

1 Vegetable Exchange

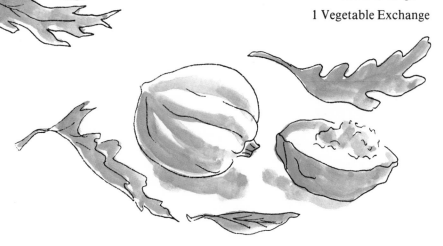

ACORN SQUASH WITH APPLESAUCE

2 acorn squash cut in half and seeded
4 teaspoons butter
2 cups applesauce, unsweetened
cinnamon
raisins

Brush each half squash with melted butter.
Bake at 350° for 45 minutes.
Fill each half with ½ cup applesauce, ¼ teaspoon cinnamon and a few raisins.
Bake 10 minutes more or until applesauce is heated through and squash is tender.

Serves 4   each: 1 Bread Exchange

1 Fruit Exchange

1 Fat Exchange

bread

Better is a dinner of herbs where love is
than a fatted ox and hatred with it.

Proverbs 15:17

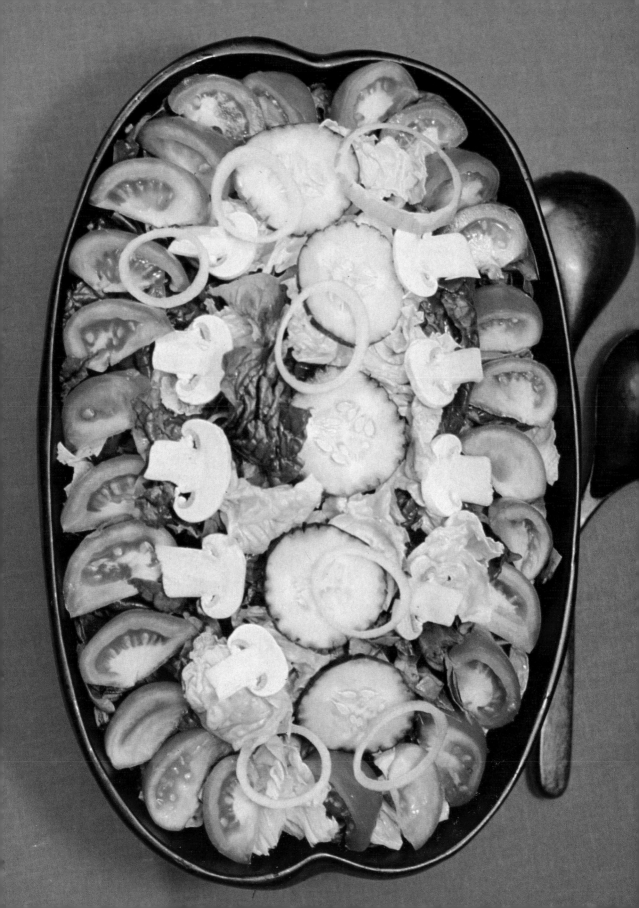

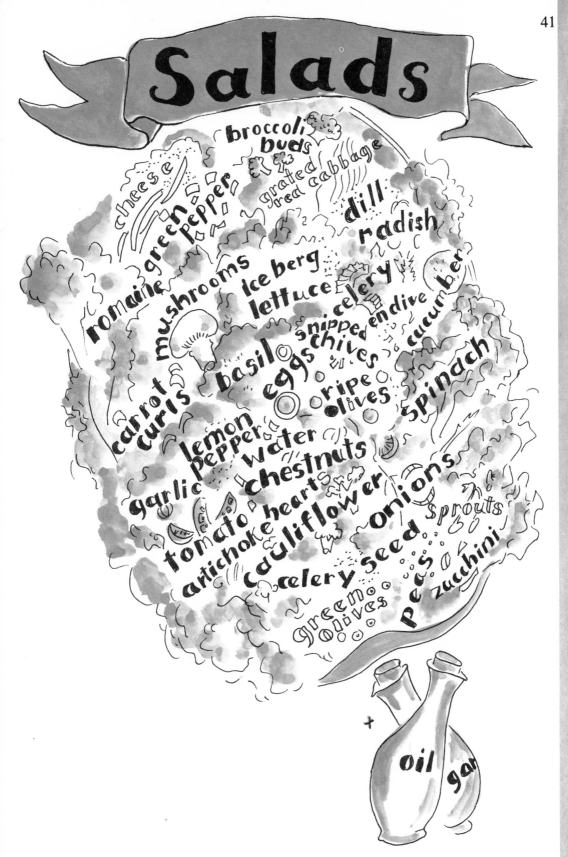

Salads

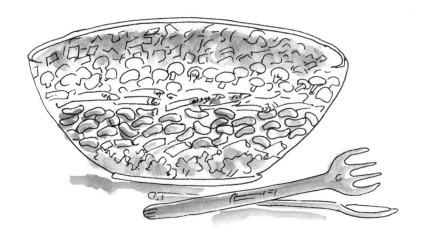

LAYERED VEGETABLE SALAD

2 cups coarsely shredded lettuce
1 (16-ounce) can whole green beans, drained
1 (15-16-ounce) can red kidney beans, drained
1 (15-ounce) can white asparagus spears,
   drained
1 (4-ounce) can button mushrooms, drained
1 (16-ounce) can sliced carrots, drained
bottled low-calorie dressing

Two hours before serving, marinate vegetables with dressing in a shallow pan.
About 15 minutes before serving: Line a
   medium glass bowl with some shredded
   lettuce; top with green beans, then with
   layers of remaining vegetables.
Serve any excess dressing separately.
Serves 12   each: 2 Vegetable Exchanges

GREEN SALAD VINAIGRETTE

2 bunches romaine
2 bunches watercress
3 cucumbers, sliced
¼ cup olive oil
¼ cup red wine vinegar
1 teaspoon salt
¼ teaspoon pepper
2 tablespoons tomato paste

Trim and wash romaine and watercress.
Tear leaves into 1-inch wide pieces.
Mix in cucumbers and put them into a salad bowl.
Cover and chill.
Combine remaining ingredients to make the dressing.
Shake well.
Let stand at room temperature.
Shake again and pour over salad.
Serves 12 each: 1 Vegetable Exchange
1 Fat Exchange

BROCCOLI-CAULIFLOWER SALAD

2 cups raw broccoli buds and stems
2 cups raw caulifflowerettes
1 teaspoon diced onions
½ cup low-calorie mayonnaise
1 teaspoon sweetener
1 teaspoon vinegar

Mix mayonnaise, sweetener and vinegar.
Toss dressing with vegetables.
Serves 8 each: 1 Vegetable Exchange
½ Fat Exchange

try different spices and herbs for variety in your salads

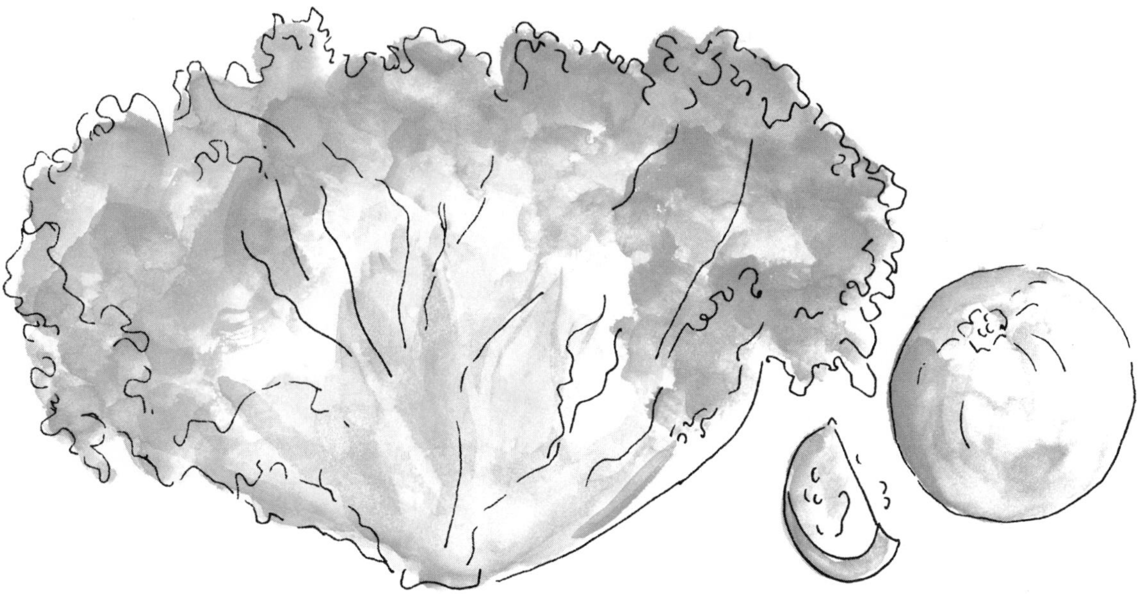

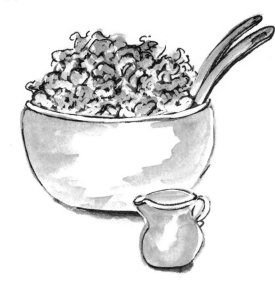

SPINACH SALAD WITH HOT SAUCE

1 pound fresh spinach
1 tablespoon vegetable oil
1 tablespoon flour
½ teaspoon salt
⅛ teaspoon pepper
2 tablespoons minced onion
¼ cup mayonnaise
3 tablespoons vinegar
½ cup water

Clean spinach, remove coarse stems, cut and
  arrange in a large salad bowl.
Put oil in frying pan and stir in flour, salt,
  pepper and onion.
Blend in mayonnaise.
Combine vinegar and water and add slowly to
  the fat mixture.
Stir until smooth.
Heat sauce until bubbly, and boil about 3
  minutes.
Do not overcook.
Pour sauce on greens and toss until well
  coated.
Serve immediately.
Serves 6   each: 1 Vegetable Exchange
                      2 Fat Exchanges

SPINACH SALAD MOLD

1 package frozen spinach (10 ounces)
1 can beef consomme
1½ envelopes gelatin
¼ cup water
2 tablespoons garlic-flavored vinegar
⅔ cup low-calorie mayonnaise
2 tablespoons lemon juice

Cook and drain spinach.
Heat consomme.
Soften gelatin in water and add lemon juice
  and vinegar.
Add hot consomme to this mixture.
Stir until gelatin is dissolved.
Chill until syrupy.
Beat with rotary beater.
Add mayonnaise and beat again.
Fold in spinach.
Pour into lightly oiled 3-cup mold.
Chill.
Serves 4   each: 1 Vegetable Exchange
                      1 Fat Exchange

SPINACH SALAD WITH BACON

1 pound raw spinach
4 slices crisp-fried bacon, crumbled
½ pound fresh mushrooms, sliced

Wash and drain spinach.
Tear into pieces.
Add bacon and mushrooms.
Toss with low-calorie Italian dressing.
Serves 6   each: 2 Vegetable Exchanges
                      1 Fat Exchange

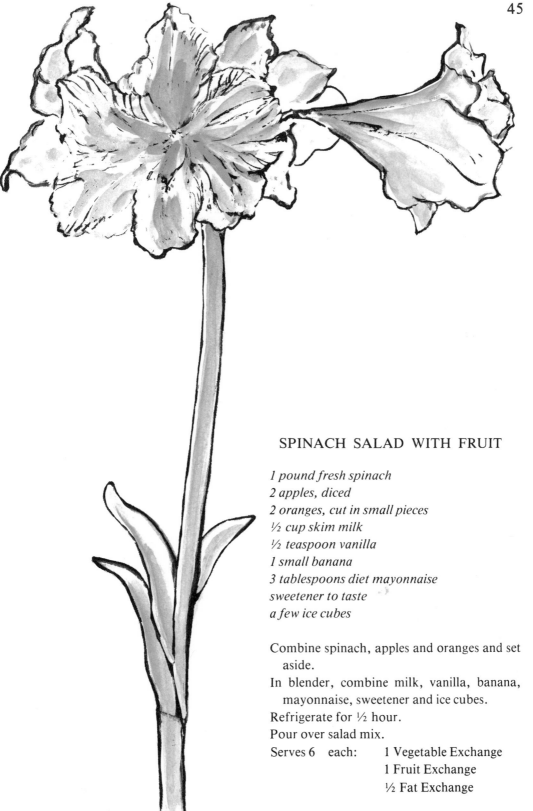

SPINACH SALAD WITH FRUIT

1 pound fresh spinach
2 apples, diced
2 oranges, cut in small pieces
½ cup skim milk
½ teaspoon vanilla
1 small banana
3 tablespoons diet mayonnaise
sweetener to taste
a few ice cubes

Combine spinach, apples and oranges and set
   aside.
In blender, combine milk, vanilla, banana,
   mayonnaise, sweetener and ice cubes.
Refrigerate for ½ hour.
Pour over salad mix.
Serves 6   each: 1 Vegetable Exchange
                    1 Fruit Exchange
                    ½ Fat Exchange

salad

CARROT-RAISIN SALAD

4 medium carrots, shredded
½ cup raisins
¼ cup low-calorie mayonnaise
¼ cup skim milk

Mix mayonnaise and skim milk together in a
  bowl.
Add remaining ingredients.
Serves 6 each: 1 Vegetable Exchange
                     1 Fruit Exchange

RICOTTA FRUIT SALAD

3 ounces Ricotta cheese
½ teaspoon vanilla extract
¼ teaspoon coconut extract
¼ cup pineapple chunks
¼ cup mandarin oranges

Whip together cheese and extracts.
Stir in pineapple and oranges.
Serve on a bed of lettuce.
Serves 1   3 Meat Exchanges
                   1 Vegetable Exchange
                   1 Fruit Exchange

CITRUS WINTER SALAD

¼ cup oil
¼ cup lemon juice
salt and pepper to taste
6 cups torn romaine
1 cup orange sections (2 medium)
1 cup grapefruit sections (1 large)
⅓ cup small green onions with tops, cut in
  1-inch slices (2 small)

In salad bowl mix oil, lemon juice, salt and
  pepper.
Combine remaining ingredients.
Toss lightly to coat, arranging fruit in pin-
  wheel pattern if desired.
Serves 4 each: 1 Vegetable Exchange
                     1 Fruit Exchange
                     1½ Fat Exchanges

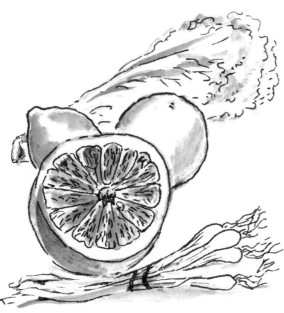

SPICY COLE SLAW

1 medium head cabbage, shredded
1 large carrot, shredded or chopped
½ small red onion, grated or chopped
¼ cup vinegar
¼ cup light corn syrup
½ teaspoon dry mustard
⅛ teaspoon parsley flakes

Mix and drain all vegetables.
In serving bowl mix vinegar, corn syrup, mustard and parsley.
Add vegetables, stir well and chill.
Serves 9   each: 1 Vegetable Exchange
                           ½ Fruit Exchange

try stirring in some unsweetened pineapple

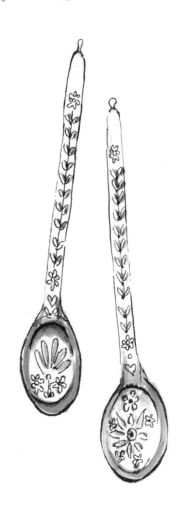

CAULIFLOWER SALAD

2 (10-ounce) packages frozen cauliflower
2 diced stalks of celery
2 tablespoons pickle relish
3 tablespoons prepared mustard
1 teaspoon parsley
artificial sweetener
½ teaspoon lemon juice
½ green pepper, chopped
4-ounce jar of mushrooms, chopped
1 tablespoon onion flakes
1 teaspoon salt
½ teaspoon Worcestershire sauce

Cook cauliflower and mash.
Combine remaining ingredients and chill before serving.
Serves 8   each: 2 Vegetable Exchanges

salad

GRATED TURNIP
AND POTATO SALAD

2 medium potatoes, cooked
3 cups grated turnips, raw
1½ teaspoons caraway seeds
3 tablespoons vinegar
3 tablespoons yogurt
salt and pepper to taste

Peel and grate potatoes and combine with re-
   maining ingredients.
Toss together lightly.
Chill and serve.
Serves 6   each: ½ Bread Exchange
                     1 Vegetable Exchange

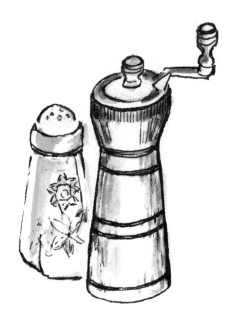

TANGY POTATO SALAD

1 tablespoon vinegar
2 tablespoons corn or safflower oil
1½ teaspoons garlic salt
1 teaspoon dillweed
¼ teaspoon pepper
8 cups boiled potatoes
¼ cup chopped pimento-stuffed olives
1½ cups sliced celery
⅓ cup sliced green onions
8 ounces low-fat plain yogurt
1 teaspoon prepared mustard

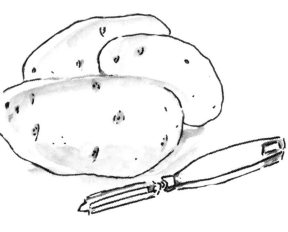

Mix the vinegar, oil, salt, dillweed and pepper
   together.
Pour this mixture over the potatoes and mix
   through gently.
Chill the potato mixture for several hours.
At serving time add olives, celery and onions.
Mix together the yogurt and mustard and fold
   this mixture into the potatoes gently and
   thoroughly.
Serves 16   each: 1 Bread Exchange

PERFECTION SALAD

2 envelopes gelatin
1 teaspoon salt
½ cup sugar
1½ cups boiling water
½ cup vinegar
2 tablespoons lemon juice
2 cups finely-shredded cabbage
1 cup chopped celery
¼ cup chopped green pepper
⅓ cup sliced, stuffed green olives

Stir gelatin, salt and sugar in boiling water
   until dissolved.
Add vinegar and lemon juice.
Chill until almost set.
Add cabbage, celery, green pepper and olives.
Pour into bread pan.
Chill until firm.
Serves 8   each: 2 Vegetable Exchanges

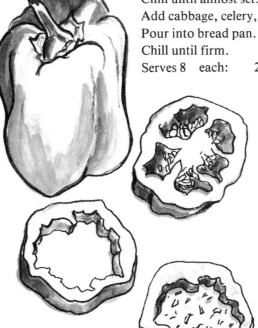

JELLIED GREEN PEPPER RINGS

4 large green peppers
1 (3-ounce) package lemon-flavored gelatin
2 cups boiling water
1 cup chopped celery
1 cup chopped carrots
1 cup shredded cabbage
1 cup drained chopped cucumbers

Cut stem end from peppers, remove seeds.
Dissolve gelatin in boiling water.
Cool until slightly thickened and add remain-
   ing ingredients.
Spoon into pepper shell and chill.
Cut each pepper crosswise into rings and
   serve on crisp lettuce.
Serves 8   each: 1 Vegetable Exchange

salad

APPLE SALAD

3 medium apples, unpeeled and cut into chunks
½ cup crushed pineapple, drained (reserve juice)
¼ cup celery, diced
2 tablespoons raisins
3 tablespoons plain yogurt
2 tablespoons mayonnaise
1 tablespoon pineapple juice
1 tablespoon lemon juice
½ teaspoon cinnamon

Combine apples, pineapple, celery and raisins.
Mix yogurt, mayonnaise, pineapple juice, lemon juice and cinnamon.
Fold mixture into dressing.
Serves 10   each: 1 Fruit Exchange
                       ½ Fat Exchange

TRUE FRUIT GELATIN

1 cup cold water
1 envelope plain gelatin
dash salt
1 cup unsweetened red grape juice
1 cup sliced strawberries or raspberries

Combine water, gelatin and salt in a saucepan.
Wait 1 minute to soften the gelatin, then heat until boiling.
When the gelatin dissolves, stir in the grape juice.
Pour into a bowl and refrigerate until syrupy.
Stir in the fruit.
Chill until set.
Serves 6   each: 1 Fruit Exchange

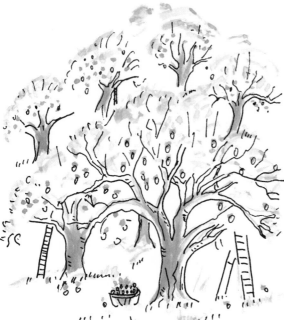

LIME-MELON MOLD

1 envelope unflavored gelatin
¼ cup cold water
1 cup hot water
½ cup lime juice
2¼ teaspoons artificial sweetener
dash salt
2 cups small melon balls

Soften gelatin over cold water; add hot water to dissolve gelatin.
Stir in lime juice, artificial sweetener and salt.
Chill until syrupy.
Fold in melon balls.
Spoon into 1-quart mold or 4 individual molds.
Chill until firm.
Serve with border of mint leaves or watercress.
Serves 4   each: 1 Fruit Exchange

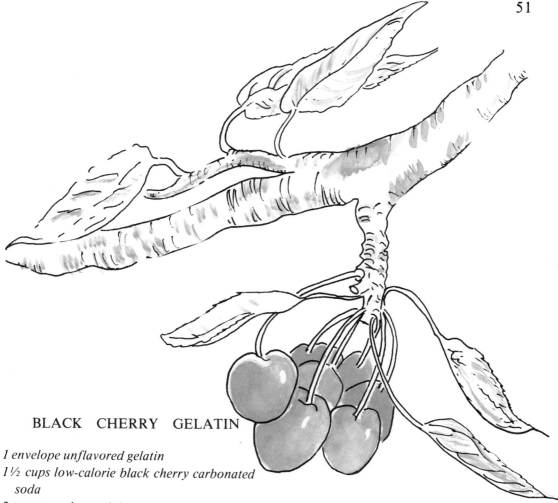

BLACK CHERRY GELATIN

1 envelope unflavored gelatin
1½ cups low-calorie black cherry carbonated
  soda
2 teaspoons lemon juice
1 teaspoon liquid sugar substitute
½ cup evaporated skim milk — very cold
½ teaspoon unflavored gelatin
½ teaspoon vanilla

Soften gelatin in ½ cup soda.
Bring to boil remaining cup of soda.
Mix with gelatin, lemon juice and sugar substitute and refrigerate until almost set.
Beat skim milk with mixer until it stands in peaks.
Slowly add gelatin.
Beat 1 minute more.
Place in gelatin mold or individual custard cups and chill.
Should be eaten same day.
Serves 2   each: ½ Milk Exchange

MOLDED PINEAPPLE SALAD

1 envelope unflavored gelatin
½ cup cold water
½ teaspoon salt
1½ cups juice from pineapple
1 can unsweetened pineapple
1 can mandarin oranges, drained and rinsed

Sprinkle gelatin over cold water in small saucepan.
Place over low heat.
Stir constantly until gelatin dissolves (about 3 minutes).
Remove from heat.
Add remaining ingredients.
Chill till firm.
Serves 9   each: 1 Fruit Exchange

salad

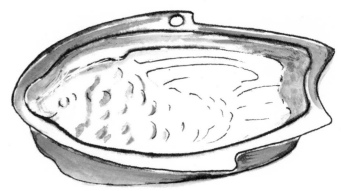

TUNA SALAD

1 (6-ounce) can tuna, drained
1 cup 2% butterfat cottage cheese
Dry onions
Parsley
Salt and pepper
5 tomatoes

Mix tuna, cottage cheese and seasonings together.
Cut a tomato on top in a star shape and scoop out middle, refill with tuna salad mixture.
Serves 5   each: 2 Meat Exchanges
1 Vegetable Exchange

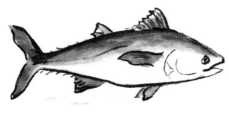

TUNA OR SALMON SALAD

6 ounces drained tuna or salmon
4 hard-boiled eggs, chopped
2 ounces cheddar cheese, grated
¼ cup onions, chopped
1 (4-ounce) can peas, drained
¼ cup celery, chopped
2 tablespoons diet salad dressing

Combine all ingredients and serve on lettuce.
Serves 6   each: 2 Meat Exchanges
1 Vegetable Exchange

TUNA-CELERY   MOLD

1 envelope unflavored gelatin
½ cup cold water
1 can cream of celery soup
¼ cup mayonnaise
1 tablespoon lemon juice
1 (7-ounce) can water-packed tuna, drained and flaked
¼ cup chopped celery
2 tablespoons chopped green pepper
1 tablespoon chopped pimento

Soften gelatin in water; stir over boiling water until gelatin is dissolved.
Blend soup, mayonnaise and lemon juice and stir into gelatin.
Chill until mixture begins to thicken.
Fold in tuna, celery, pepper and pimento.
Pour into 3-cup mold.
Chill until firm; unmold; serve on crisp salad greens.
Serves 4   each: 2 Meat Exchanges
½ Bread Exchange
1 Vegetable Exchange
2 Fat Exchanges

TUNA FRUIT SALAD

2 medium unpeeled apples
4 cups lettuce, torn
1 (9¼-ounce) can water-packed tuna
1 cup seedless green grapes
½ cup low-calorie mayonnaise
1 tablespoon lemon juice
¼ teaspoon salt

APPLE AND TUNA SALAD

1 (7-ounce) can water-packed tuna, drained
1 medium-size tart apple, cored and chopped
1 stalk celery, chopped
3 tablespoons low-calorie mayonnaise
2 tablespoons lemon juice
1 tablespoon minced onion
¼ teaspoon dillweed
salt and pepper to taste

Cut apples in ½-inch cubes and toss together
   with torn lettuce, tuna (drained and flaked)
   and grapes.
Cover and chill.
Combine mayonnaise, lemon juice and salt;
   toss with tuna mixture.
Serves 4   each: 2 Meat Exchanges
                      1 Vegetable Exchange
                      1 Fruit Exchange
                      2 Fat Exchanges

Combine all ingredients in medium bowl.
   Chill.
Serve on salad greens.
Serves 2   each: 3 Meat Exchanges
                      1 Vegetable Exchange
                      1 Fruit Exchange
                      ½ Fat Exchange
Note: For a cold summer salad, add diced,
   cooked beets.

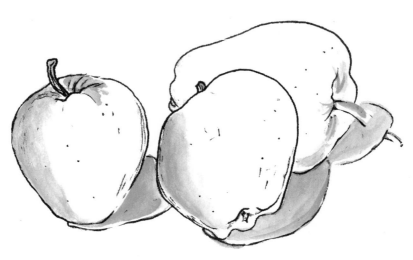

salad

54

CRAB SALAD

1 cup crab meat, drained and flaked
1 cup chopped celery
2 hard-boiled eggs, chopped
1 tablespoon grated onion
1 teaspoon lemon juice
2 tablespoons low-calorie mayonnaise
Salt and pepper to taste

Combine ingredients, mixing thoroughly.
Chill for 1 hour.
Serve on lettuce with egg wedges and paprika
   or use as a sandwich.
Serves 3   each: 3 Meat Exchanges
                       1 Fat Exchange

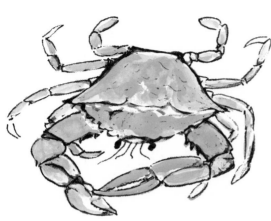

SOUFFLE TUNA ASPIC

1 envelope unflavored gelatin
¼ cup cold water
¾ cup hot chicken broth
¾ cup cold water
1½ teaspoons lemon juice
2 (7-ounce) cans water-packed tuna
¼ cup chopped green pepper
¼ cup finely chopped celery

Add gelatin and lemon juice to ¼ cup cold
   water to soften.
Add hot chicken broth and dissolve com-
   pletely.
Set until firm.
Place in blender with cold water and blend
   until frothy.
Pour into bowl and let stand until it starts to
   thicken.
Fold in other ingredients.
Pour into mold.
Chill overnight.
Unmold on a bed of shredded lettuce.
Serves 6   each: 2 Meat Exchanges
                   ½ Vegetable Exchange
May garnish with slices of hard-cooked eggs
   (optional).

SHRIMP SALAD

1 pound shrimp, cooked or 10 ounces, canned
1 cup chopped celery
2 hard-cooked eggs, chopped
3 tablespoons diced dill pickle
½ cup low-fat plain yogurt
½ teaspoon Worcestershire sauce
¾ teaspoon salt
¼ teaspoon pepper
lettuce

Chill shrimp and if large, cut in halves or
 quarters.
Toss together shrimp, celery, eggs and pickle.
Combine yogurt, Worcestershire sauce and
 seasonings; add to shrimp mixture.
Serve on crisp lettuce or salad greens.
Garnish top with shrimp and egg.
Serves 3   each: 3 Meat Exchanges

Note: If using canned shrimp, decrease salt to
 ¼ teaspoon.

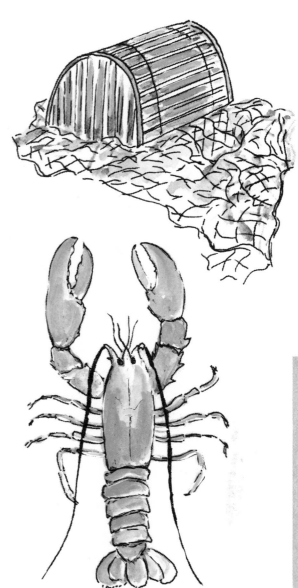

SEAFOOD SALAD

1 cup flaked cooked sea food (crab-meat,
 shrimp, lobster, tuna, salmon)
½ teaspoon lemon juice
½ teaspoon finely chopped onion
½ cup diced celery
2 tablespoons mayonnaise
½ cup lettuce in small pieces

If canned seafood is used, drain off oil.
Lightly mix ingredients in order.
Chill thoroughly.
Just before serving, toss with mayonnaise to
 moisten.
Serves 4   each: 2 Meat Exchanges
                      1 Vegetable Exchange
                      1 Fat Exchange
Garnish with lemon wedges or hard-cooked
egg slices (optional).

salad

56

CHICKEN AND POTATO SALAD

8 ounces cold chicken, diced
2 stalks celery, diced
4 (2-inch) cooked potatoes, diced
salt and pepper to taste
4 tablespoons low-calorie mayonnaise

Mix well and serve on a bed of lettuce.
Serves 4   each: 2 Meat Exchanges
                      1 Vegetable Exchange

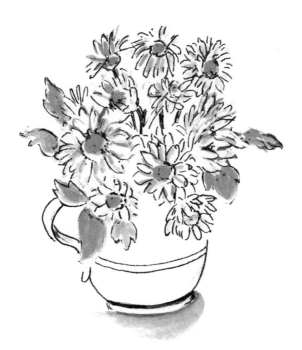

JELLIED   CHICKEN   LOAF

1½ tablespoons unflavored gelatin
½ cup cold water
1¼ cups chicken bouillon (prepared)
1½ cups chopped cooked chicken
¾ cup whole cranberry sauce, low-calorie

Sprinkle 1 tablespoon gelatin on ¼ cup cold
  water.
Heat chicken bouillon to boiling.
Add softened gelatin; stir until dissolved.
Chill until mixture begins to thicken; fold in
  chicken.

Pour into 4-cup loaf pan.
Sprinkle remaining gelatin over ¼ cup cold
  water.
Dissolve in hot cranberry sauce.
Chill until partially thickened.
Pour cranberry sauce over chicken loaf; chill
  until firm.
Unmold on platter.
Serves 6   each: 2 Meat Exchanges
                      1 Fruit Exchange

STEAK-MUSHROOM SALAD

2 ounces sliced leftover steak
½ cup sliced mushrooms, raw
½ small red onion, thinly sliced
1 cup shredded romaine
2 tablespoons low-calorie French dressing
¼ teaspoon salt or garlic salt
fresh ground pepper

Toss ingredients together.
Serves 1   2 Meat Exchanges
                    2 Vegetable Exchanges
                    1 Fat Exchange

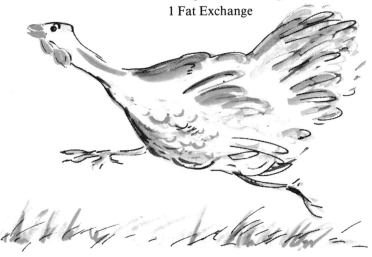

TURKEY AND APPLE SALAD

2 cups diced, cooked turkey or chicken
2 small apples
1 stalk celery
½ cup low-calorie mayonnaise
¼ cup raisins
1 tablespoon lemon juice
Salt to taste
Curry powder (optional)
Salad greens

Cut up apples and celery.
Mix all ingredients except salad greens.
Chill before serving.
Serve on salad greens.
Serves 8   each: 2 Meat Exchanges
                      1 Fruit Exchange

salad

LOW CALORIE RANCH DRESSING

1 cup buttermilk
1 tablespoon garlic salt
½ teaspoon parsley flakes
½ teaspoon onion flakes
*¼ teaspoon monosodium glutamate (op-
tional)*
⅛ teaspoon pepper
2 teaspoons red wine vinegar

Combine all ingredients.
Keeps several days in the refrigerator.
¼ cup = ¼ Milk Exchange

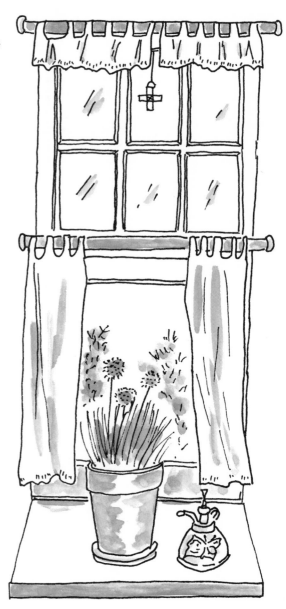

PINEAPPLE VINEGAR
SALAD DRESSING

½ cup unsweetened pineapple juice
½ cup vinegar
¼ teaspoon dry mustard
⅛ teaspoon sweet basil
⅛ teaspoon paprika
2-3 pinches garlic powder
Salt and pepper to taste

Add vinegar to pineapple juice, beating constantly.
Add remaining ingredients.
Keeps well for about a week in the refrigerator.
1 tablespoon is a Free Exchange.

*a windowsill
herb garden~
chives and parsley~
a wonderful addition
to your kitchen*

COTTAGE CHEESE DELIGHT DRESSING

1 (12-ounce) carton cream-style cottage cheese
2 tablespoons skim milk
½ teaspoon salt

Blend all ingredients in electric blender till light and fluffy (or beat 5 minutes with electric beater).

Fluffed like this, cottage cheese makes a dressing for tomato slices or fruit.

¼ cup = 1 Meat Exchange

FRENCH DRESSING

½ cup oil
½ cup lemon juice or vinegar
Paprika
1 teaspoon catsup
½ teaspoon salt
½ teaspoon dry mustard
½ teaspoon Worcestershire sauce
1 clove of garlic

Shake well in a jar and chill.
Each tablespoon equals 1 Fat Exchange

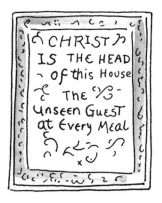

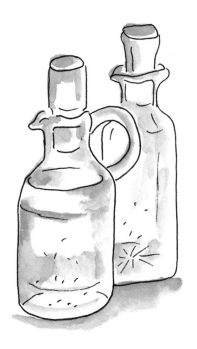

YOGURT SALAD DRESSING
(or dip)

½ cup low-fat plain yogurt
¼ cup low-calorie mayonnaise
1½ teaspoons ranch dry dressing mix
1 teaspoon Italian dry dressing mix
1 teaspoon lemon juice
½ teaspoon onion juice

Combine all ingredients. Mix until smooth.
2 tablespoons = ½ Fat Exchange

salad

Test your servants for ten days; let us be given vegetables to eat and water to drink.

Daniel 1:12

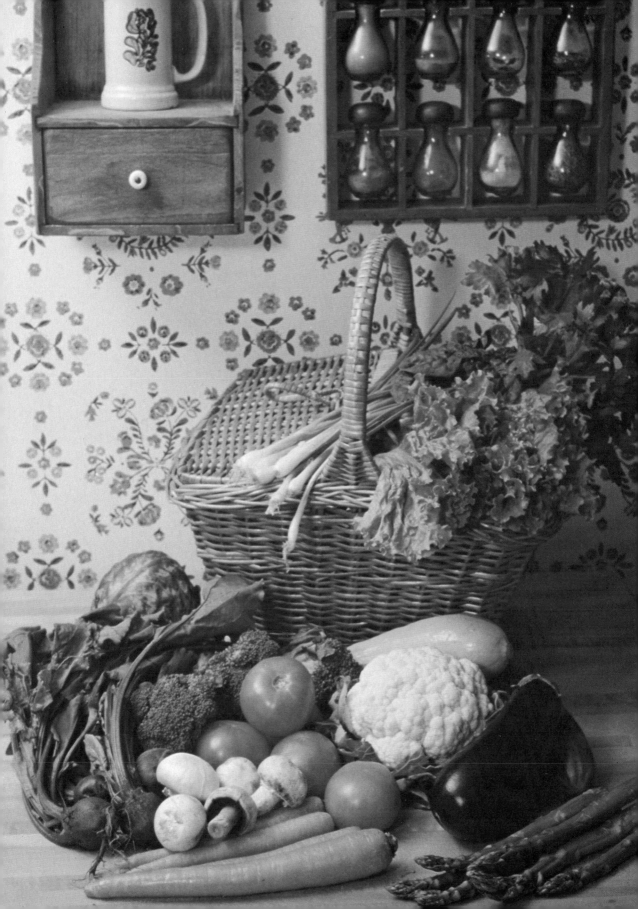

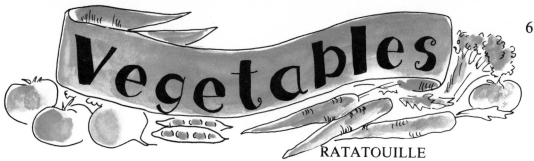

RATATOUILLE

1 small eggplant
2 small zucchini
1 large onion
1 large green pepper
½ cup olive oil
1 clove garlic, chopped
2 tomatoes, chopped
3 tablespoons parsley, chopped
½ teaspoon salt
¼ teaspoon pepper
1 teaspoon leaf oregano, crumbled
1 teaspoon leaf basil, crumbled

Cut eggplant into ½-inch thick slices, then cut into ½-inch cubes.

Cut zucchini into ¼-inch slices; slice onion thinly.

Cut green pepper into ¼-inch strips.

In a skillet, saute eggplant cubes in 2 tablespoons of oil until lightly browned (about 5 minutes).

Remove to large saucepan or Dutch oven.

Add 1 tablespoon more oil to skillet.

Saute zucchini until tender; remove to saucepan.

Add remaining oil to skillet; saute onion, green pepper and garlic until tender, then combine with eggplant and zucchini in saucepan.

Add tomatoes, parsley, salt, pepper, oregano and basil.

Stir gently to mix.

Simmer mixture, covered, over low heat for 15 minutes.

Remove cover and simmer 10 minutes longer, or until most of the free liquid has cooked away.

Add additional seasoning if you wish.

Serves 8   each: 1 Vegetable Exchange
1½ Fat Exchanges

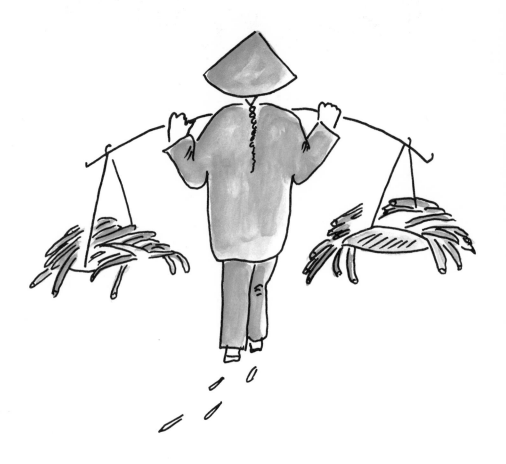

MARINATED ASPARAGUS

Cook 1 pound of asparagus until almost
  done.
Drain and pour ½ cup low-calorie Italian
  dressing over asparagus.
Refrigerate.
Serve cold; garnish with pimento.
Serves 4   each: 1 Vegetable Exchange

CHINESE ASPARAGUS

Cut 1 pound of asparagus diagonally in ½-¼
  inch slices.
Heat 1 teaspoon oil in heavy skillet.
Add asparagus and sprinkle with salt.
Cover pan and cook 3 minutes or until fork
  tender.
Serve topped with slivered almonds (optional).

Serves 4   each: 1 Vegetable Exchange

PICKLED BEETS

1 (16-ounce) can beets, drained
½ cup vinegar
1 cup water
½ stick cinnamon
¼ teaspoon salt
artificial sweetener equal to ⅓ cup sugar
4 whole cloves

Combine all ingredients except beets.
Simmer 10 minutes.
Add beets and simmer 5 minutes.
Pour into pint jars and refrigerate when cool.
Serves 4   each: 1 Vegetable Exchange

COMPANY BEETS

1 tablespoon brown sugar
1 tablespoon cornstarch
¼ teaspoon salt
1 cup pineapple chunks with juice
1 tablespoon butter
1 tablespoon lemon juice
2 cups drained, diced beets

Combine sugar, cornstarch and salt in saucepan.
Add pineapple with juice. Cook, stirring
   constantly, until thick and bubbly. Add remaining ingredients and heat through.
Serves 4   each: 1 Vegetable Exchange
                     1 Fruit Exchange
                     ½ Fat Exchange

GLAZED TURNIPS

12 ounces small white turnips, peeled if
   necessary (about 1½ cups)
½ teaspoon salt
water (about 1 inch in bottom of saucepan)
2 tablespoons apple juice
1 tablespoon butter

Boil turnips in salted water until tender and
   water has boiled off.
Add apple juice and continue boiling (uncovered) until juice has been absorbed.
Add butter and shake pot constantly, turning
   the turnips until all are coated and shiny
   golden brown.
Serves 4   each: 1 Vegetable Exchange
                     ½ Fat Exchange

BEETS AND BEET TOPS

1 dozen tiny fresh beets with tops
1½ teaspoons salt
3 tablespoons vinegar

Wash beets and tops.
Cook in covered pan until tender.
Add salt and vinegar.
Serves 4   each: 1 Vegetable Exchange

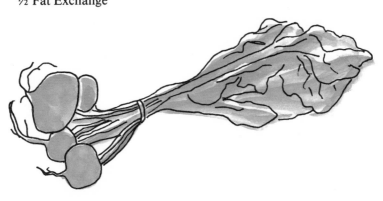

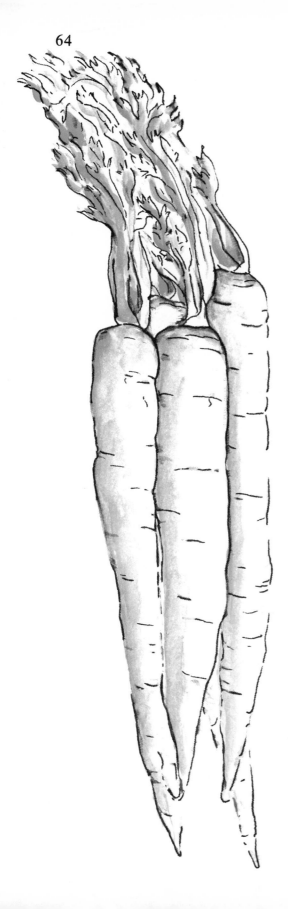

LEMON   CARROTS

2 pounds carrots
⅓ cup melted butter
1 tablespoon sugar
1 tablespoon minced parsley
1 teaspoon paprika
1 lemon

Cut carrots into strips or slices.
Cook in small amount of water until barely
   tender. Drain water.
Add butter, sugar, parsley, paprika and juice
   of lemon.
Saute the carrots for 5 minutes.

Serves 10   each: 1 Vegetable Exchange
                       ½ Fat Exchange

ORANGE-DILLED   CARROTS

2 cups sliced, pared carrots
1 teaspoon salt
2 teaspoons butter or margarine
½ teaspoon dill weed
1 cup fresh orange sections or bite-size pieces
½ teaspoon grated orange rind

Place carrots in medium saucepan with 1 cup
   water and ½ teaspoon salt.
Bring to boil, cover and simmer for 15 minutes, or until tender; drain.
Add ½ teaspoon salt and remaining ingredients.
Stir over low heat for 1 or 2 minutes.

Serves 4   each: 1 Vegetable Exchange
                      ½ Fruit Exchange

SAUTEED CARROTS

8 carrots, diced or thinly sliced
2 teaspoons oil
1 tablespoon water
1 teaspoon salt

Put all ingredients in heavy pan; cover.
Heat quickly, then reduce heat.
Cook 10-15 minutes.
Serves 4   each: 1 Vegetable Exchange
                            ½ Fat Exchange

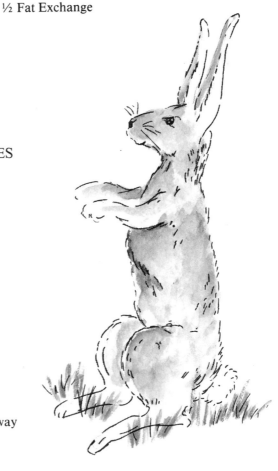

PARSLEY CARROTS & POTATOES

1½ teaspoons salt
1 cup water
2 cups thinly sliced carrots
2 cups thinly sliced potatoes
¼ cup minced onion
2 tablespoons margarine or butter
½ cup chopped or snipped parsley
1 teaspoon caraway seeds
⅛ teaspoon pepper

Bring salted water to boil in saucepan.
Add carrots, potatoes and onion.
Cover and cook until tender.
Drain.
Lightly toss in margarine, parsley, caraway
   seeds and pepper until blended.
Serves 4   each: 1 Bread Exchange
                           1 Vegetable Exchange
                           1 Fat Exchange

66

BRUSSELS SPROUTS IN MUSHROOM SAUCE

1 pound Brussels sprouts
1 can mushroom soup
½ cup skim evaporated milk
1 teaspoon salt

Parboil Brussels sprouts for 10 minutes.
Mix soup and milk and heat.
Add the Brussels sprouts and simmer until tender, about 10-12 minutes.
(Good with broccoli also).

Serves 4   each: ½ Bread Exchange
1 Vegetable Exchange
1 Milk Exchange
1 Fat Exchange

CABBAGE MEDLEY

1 large cabbage, sliced
2 shredded carrots
1 medium diced potato
1 diced onion
1 teaspoon chicken or beef bouillon

Add all ingredients to 1 cup of boiling water.
Cook for about 8-10 minutes.
Serves 8   each: ½ Bread Exchange
1 Vegetable Exchange

CABBAGE IN BACON

6 cups cabbage, coarsely chopped
4 slices bacon, cooked
½ teaspoon salt

Cook bacon in skillet.
Remove bacon to paper towel.
Remove all bacon fat from skillet except 2 tablespoons.
Place cabbage in skillet and cook covered 5-6 minutes.
Sprinkle crumbled bacon over top.
Serves 8   each: 1 Vegetable Exchange
½ Fat Exchange

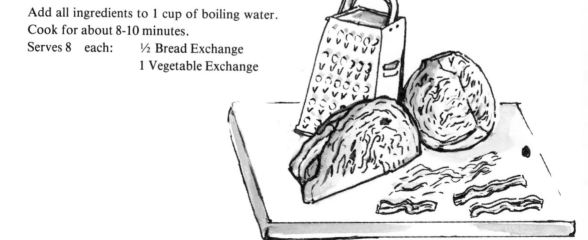

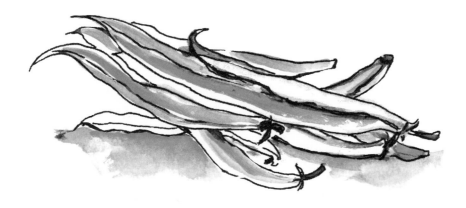

GREEN BEANS SCANDIA

1 can cut green beans (1 pound)
2 chicken bouillon cubes
2 tablespoons butter or margarine
1 tablespoon sugar
dash pepper
1 tablespoon cornstarch
1 tablespoon cold water
3-4 tablespoons vinegar
2 cups chopped cabbage

Drain liquid from beans into saucepan.

Add next 4 ingredients.

Heat to boiling, stirring constantly.

Stir cornstarch into cold water and add to above mixture.

Cook, stirring, until mixture thickens and is clear.

Add vinegar and cabbage.

Bring to a boil, simmer covered about 5 minutes or until tender.

Add beans. Reheat.

Serves 4   each: ½ Bread Exchange
2 Vegetable Exchanges
1 Fat Exchange

GREEN BEANS PROVENCAL

¼ cup oil
¾ cup sliced onions
1 clove minced garlic
1 teaspoon salt
½ teaspoon oregano
½ cup sliced green pepper
½ cup chopped celery
1 cup canned tomatoes
¼ teaspoon pepper
1 bay leaf
¼ cup water
2 (16-ounce) cans drained green beans

Heat oil and saute onions 5 minutes.

Add all ingredients except green beans.

Bring to a boil, reduce heat to low and cook for 10 minutes.

Add beans.

Heat 5 minutes.

Serves 6   each: 2 Vegetable Exchanges
2 Fat Exchanges

68

FRENCH ALMOND GREEN BEANS

2 cans French style green beans
1 teaspoon chicken bouillon
dash pepper
mushrooms, optional
¼ cup slivered almonds

Drain ½ of liquid off beans.
Add bouillon, pepper and mushrooms.
Heat, drain, and add almonds.
Serves 8   each: 1 Vegetable Exchange
                              ½ Fat Exchange

*add some
onion salt
to water
when
cooking
beans*

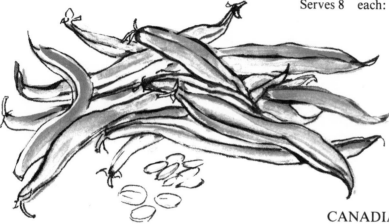

CANADIAN GREEN BEANS

1 pound fresh green beans or
1 (9-ounce) package frozen beans
¼ cup boiling water
1 tablespoon diet margarine
½ cup finely diced Canadian bacon
1 clove garlic, minced
½ teaspoon salt
¼ teaspoon pepper
1 tomato, cut in wedges

CHEESY BEAN CASSEROLE

1 can green beans
½ cup skim milk
2 ounces American cheese
1 slice bread, crumbled

Warm beans. Drain off liquid and put beans
  into 1-quart casserole.
Heat milk, add cheese and bread crumbs, stirring until cheese melts.
Pour over green beans and bake for 15 minutes at 350°
Serves 4   each: 1 Meat Exchange
                              1 Vegetable Exchange

Cook green beans in the water until they are
  tender; drain.
Melt the margarine in a non-stick skillet and
  saute the bacon and garlic until they are
  brown.
Add the beans, salt and pepper to the skillet,
  and top with the tomato wedges.
Cover the pan and heat the contents through.
Serves 4   each: 1 Meat Exchange
                              2 Vegetable Exchanges

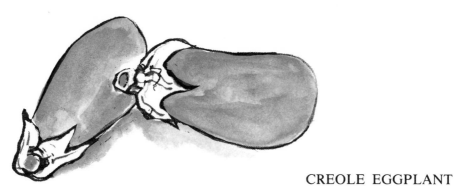

CREOLE EGGPLANT

1 small eggplant, peeled and diced
1 pint tomato juice
¼ onion, diced
¼ green pepper, optional
salt and pepper to taste

Place all ingredients in saucepan and simmer
about 25 minutes until eggplant is tender.
Serves 8   each: 1 Vegetable Exchange

CAULIFLOWER ITALIANO

1 tablespoon chopped onion
1 small clove garlic, crushed
2 tablespoons low-calorie Italian dressing
3 cups small fresh cauliflowerets
2 tablespoons chopped green pepper
1 cup cherry tomatoes, halved
½ teaspoon salt
⅛ teaspoon dried basil, crushed

In 8-inch skillet cook onion and garlic in
salad dressing until tender.
Add cauliflowerets and ¼ cup water.
Cook covered over low heat 10 minutes.
Add green pepper; cook until cauliflower is
tender, about 5 minutes.
Stir in remaining ingredients.
Cook until heated through.
Serves 8   each: 1 Vegetable Exchange

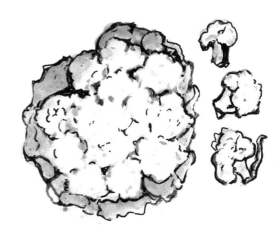

STIR FRY VEGETABLES

1 cup broccoli
1 cup onions
½ pound mushrooms
½ cup water chestnuts

Add any vegetables you like, sliced thinly.
Use 1 package of chicken broth mix with a
 little water.
Stir-fry until tender.
Serves 6   each: 1 Vegetable Exchange

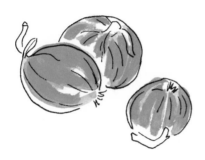

BAKED TOMATOES AND ONIONS

18 small onions
3½ cups whole canned tomatoes
1 teaspoon salt
1 teaspoon basil
⅛ teaspoon pepper
1 tablespoon brown sugar
¼ cup bread crumbs
2 tablespoons butter

Peel onions; cook in boiling salted water for
 20 minutes; drain.
Combine tomatoes, salt, pepper, sugar and
 basil, and turn into 1½-quart casserole.
Add onions.
Sprinkle with bread crumbs and dot with
 butter.
Bake uncovered at 350° for 35-40 minutes.
Serves 8   each: 1 Bread Exchange
                                2 Vegetable Exchanges
                                1 Fat Exchange

MUSHROOM COCKTAIL

Fresh mushrooms, cut up
Shredded lettuce
Seafood cocktail sauce

Wash mushrooms and sprinkle with a little
 lemon juice.
Let stand 1 hour in refrigerator.
Put in dish on top of shredded lettuce.
Top with seafood cocktail sauce.
Chill in refrigerator before serving.
½ cup serving = 1 Vegetable Exchange

STEWED ONIONS

6 onions
1 cup beef bouillon
1 teaspoon butter-flavored salt

Slice 6 onions into rings.
Cook in bouillon and salt until tender and
 liquid is reduced.
Serves 6   each: 1 Vegetable Exchange

BAKED ONIONS

4 medium onions
diet Italian salad dressing
paprika

Peel onions, and cut in half.
Grease a baking dish with diet Italian salad
 dressing.
Put onions in baking dish and pour 1 tea-
 spoon dressing on top of each half.
Sprinkle with paprika.
Bake at 350° for 30-45 minutes.
Serves 4   each: 1 Vegetable Exchange

ROMANIAN VEGETABLE POTPOURRI

2 medium onions, sliced thinly
2 large cloves garlic, crushed
2 tablespoons olive oil
1 medium eggplant cut in ½-inch cubes
2 medium tomatoes, peeled and diced
1 medium green pepper, cut in strips
1 small yellow squash, cut in 1½-inch strips
1 medium potato, diced
1 cup chicken broth
½ teaspoon salt
¼ teaspoon fresh ground pepper
1 tomato, chopped (optional)

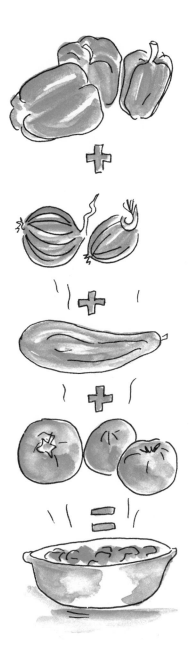

In Dutch oven saute onions and garlic in hot oil until tender, about 5-7 minutes.

Stir in eggplant, diced tomatoes, green pepper, squash, potato, broth, salt and pepper.

Bring to boil.

Cover and simmer, stirring occasionally, 20-25 minutes or until vegetables are tender and liquid has been absorbed.

Serve warm, at room temperature or chilled.

Garnish with chopped tomato.

Serves 5   each:　　1 Bread Exchange
　　　　　　　　　　1 Vegetable Exchange
　　　　　　　　　　1 Fat Exchange

VEGETABLE GOULASH

3 peppers, cut up
2 onions, sliced
1 large summer squash, cubed
3 red tomatoes, cut up
salt and pepper

Saute peppers, onions and cubed squash until soft, using as little oil as possible (1 tablespoon).

Add cut-up tomatoes.

Simmer 15 or 20 minutes in large frying pan.

Serves 4   each:　　2 Vegetable Exchanges
　　　　　　　　　　1 Fat Exchange

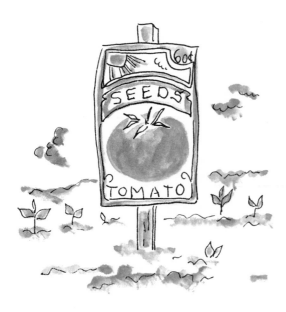

STUFFED TOMATOES

6 large, firm, ripe tomatoes
1 (4-ounce) can sliced mushrooms
1 (6-ounce) package stuffing mix, chicken
   flavor
½ cup grated cheddar or American cheese

Cut thin slice from stem end of each tomato.
Remove seeds and pulp, leaving a shell about
½ inch thick; reserve about ¾ cup pulp.
Drain mushrooms, reserving liquid.
Combine tomato pulp and mushroom liquid
   and add water to make 1¾ cups.
Prepare stuffing mix as directed on package,
   using measured liquid; add mushrooms
   with the stuffing crumbs.
Spoon stuffing into tomato shells.
Place in shallow baking dish and sprinkle
   with cheese.
Bake at 350° for 30 minutes.
Serves 6   each: ½ Bread Exchange
                   1 Vegetable Exchange
                   1½ Fat Exchanges

SCALLOPED TOMATOES

¼ cup margarine
1 small onion, chopped
2 cups fresh bread crumbs
1 teaspoon salt
½ teaspoon basil
¼ teaspoon pepper
2 (14½-ounce) cans sliced baby tomatoes
4 teaspoons sugar

About 40 minutes before serving:
Cook onion in margarine over medium heat,
   until tender, about 5 minutes.
Stir in bread crumbs, salt, basil and pepper.
In 1½-quart casserole, place ¼ of tomato
   slices and their liquid; sprinkle with 1 tea-
   spoon sugar and ¼ of the onion mixture.
Repeat layering 3 more times.
Bake at 375° for 20-30 minutes.
Serves 8   each: 1 Bread Exchange
                   1 Vegetable Exchange
                   2 Fat Exchanges

MARINATED VEGETABLE
MEDLEY

1 can V-8 juice (24-ounce)
½ cup vegetable oil
¼ cup vinegar
2 cups cauliflowerettes
1 cup thin-sliced carrots
1 cup cubes or strips of zucchini
½ cup green pepper squares

Mix juice, oil and vinegar for marinade.
Mix vegetables.
Pour marinade over and chill.
Other favorite vegetables can be substituted if
   desired.
Serves 8   each: 2 Vegetable Exchanges
                   1 Fat Exchange

TOMATO ZUCCHINI CASSEROLE

1 pound can whole tomatoes
2 medium zucchini, thinly sliced
1 medium onion, chopped
¼ stick butter
¼ teaspoon salt
¾ cup grated Swiss cheese

Saute onion in butter until lightly colored.
Add sliced zucchini and cook just until tender.
Add tomatoes, salt and pepper.
Bring to boil.
Remove from heat.
Place in 2-quart casserole or heat-resistant serving dish.
Sprinkle cheese over top.
Place under broiler until cheese melts and browns.
Serves 8   each: 1 Vegetable Exchange
                    1 Fat Exchange

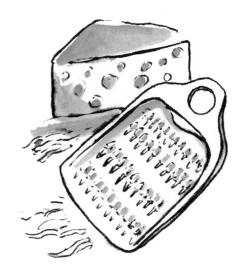

vegetable

ZUCCHINI WITH GARLIC

1 zucchini unpeeled, sliced into ¼-inch rounds
1 clove garlic, split
¼ teaspoon salt
⅛ teaspoon pepper
⅛ teaspoon lemon extract
pinch of oregano
fresh or canned tomatoes may be added

Put all ingredients into a heavy pan.
Cook tightly covered over very low heat for 15 minutes or until zucchini is tender.
Remove garlic before serving.
Serves 2   each: 1 Vegetable Exchange

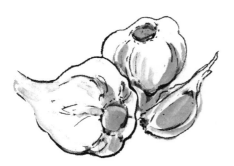

SUMMER SQUASH

2 medium summer squash
1 tomato, cut up
dash basil
2 tablespoons chopped onions
2 tablespoons Parmesan cheese

Combine all ingredients and simmer until tender (10-15 mins.).
Serves 6   each: 1 Vegetable Exchange

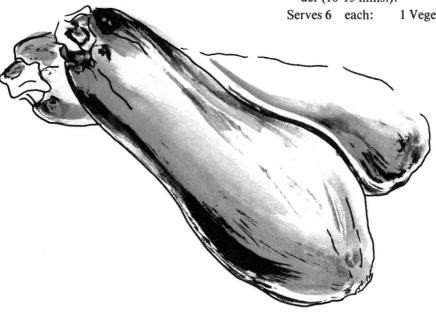

BAKED SPICED SQUASH

½-1 pound yellow squash
salt to taste
2 tablespoons onion flakes
½ cup milk
Parmesan cheese (optional)

Slice squash, put in pie plate.
Add onion flakes over this.
Cover with milk.
Sprinkle salt over all.
Top with Parmesan cheese if desired.
Bake at 350° for 40 minutes.
Serves 4   each: 1 Vegetable Exchange
                      ½ Milk Exchange

ZUCCHINI WITH TOMATO AND CHEESE

3 cups zucchini
1 onion, chopped
1 tablespoon vegetable oil
1 teaspoon salt
½ cup shredded cheese
1 cup canned tomatoes

Brown zucchini and onion in oil, cover and simmer 10 minutes.
Add rest of ingredients and heat until cheese melts.
Serves 8   each: 1 Vegetable Exchange
                      ¾ Fat Exchange

ZUCCHINI CASSEROLE

3 medium zucchini
2 eggs
½ tablespoon dried, minced onion
salt and pepper to taste
½ cup shredded cheddar cheese
2 teaspoons chopped green chilies (optional)
⅔ cup cracker or bread crumbs

Boil or steam zucchini which has been cut into ½-inch slices.

When tender, drain off water and mash thoroughly.

Add remaining ingredients until well mixed.

Put mix in buttered 1-quart casserole dish.

Top with additional grated cheese, if desired.

Bake at 350° for 20-30 minutes.

Serves 6   each: ½ Meat Exchange
                         2 Vegetable Exchanges
                         1 Fat Exchange

SKILLET ZUCCHINI

4 large zucchini
2 tablespoons margarine
1 small onion, minced
1 envelope chicken bouillon or
1 tablespoon chicken stock base
1 teaspoon salt

Cut each zucchini in half lengthwise, then crosswise.

Using a 10-inch skillet, saute onion in margarine.

Add zucchini, cut side down; cook 10 minutes or until under-side is golden.

Meanwhile in measuring cup, mix well ½ cup hot water, bouillon and salt.

Reduce heat to low; pour mix over zucchini, cover and simmer 10 minutes.

Serves 8   each: 1 Vegetable Exchange
                         ½ Fat Exchange

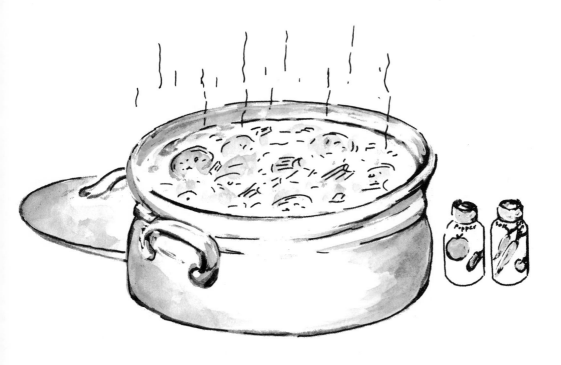

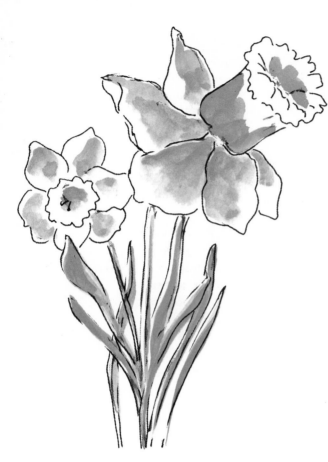

SPINACH LOAF

1 box frozen spinach
2 tablespoons butter
3 tablespoons flour
1 teaspoon salt
1 cup skim milk
2 eggs

Add milk to butter, flour and salt to make a
  cream sauce.
Add slightly beaten eggs.
Combine all ingredients and pour into but-
  tered casserole.
Bake at 350° for 35-40 minutes.
Serves 4   each: ½ Bread Exchange
                      1 Vegetable Exchange
                      1 Fat Exchange

SPINACH WITH BLUE CHEESE

10 ounces spinach, fresh or frozen
1 bouillon cube (beef)
1 can evaporated skim milk (13-ounce)
1 tablespoon crumbled blue cheese
⅛ teaspoon onion salt
salt and pepper to taste
3 teaspoons vinegar
1 tablespoon Italian cheese, grated

Cook spinach in prepared bouillon. Drain
  and keep hot.
Heat milk with blue cheese, seasoned with
  onion, salt and pepper.
Into casserole dish place hot, fluffed spinach.
Sprinkle with vinegar.
Pour hot milk mixture over.
Sprinkle with Italian cheese.
Serve immediately.
If returned to oven it will separate slowly.
Serves 8   each: 1 Vegetable Exchange
                    ½ Milk Exchange

SCALLOPED SPINACH

1 (10-ounce) package frozen spinach, cooked
  and drained
1 tablespoon finely-chopped onion
2 beaten eggs
½ cup skim milk
½ cup shredded sharp cheddar cheese
½ cup buttered bread crumbs

Combine all ingredients except bread crumbs.
Put in a casserole dish and top with crumbs.
Bake at 350° about 20-30 minutes or until
  knife inserted comes out clean.
Serves 4   each: 1 Meat Exchange
                       ½ Bread Exchange
                       1 Vegetable Exchange
                       ½ Milk Exchange

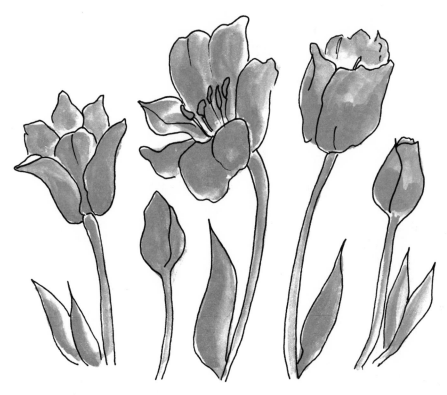

SPINACH BAKE

2 (10-ounce) packages frozen spinach, cooked
    and drained
2 tablespoons margarine
1 tablespoon chicken bouillon powder or 1
    cube crushed
¼ teaspoon garlic powder
2 tablespoons cornstarch
1 cup skim milk
pepper to taste
¼-½ cup grated cheese

Dissolve cornstarch in milk.
Melt margarine with bouillon and garlic; add
    milk to mixture and cook until thick.
Stir in grated cheese.
Combine with spinach.
Bake at 350° for 20 minutes or more.
Serves 6   each: 1 Vegetable Exchange
                     ½ Milk Exchange
                     1 Fat Exchange

SOUTHERN SPINACH

1 (10-ounce) package frozen, chopped
    spinach
1 (8-ounce) can grapefruit sections
½ teaspoon salt
1 teaspoon lemon juice
cinnamon
pepper

About 20 minutes before serving: cook spin-
    ach according to package directions but
    substitute juice drained from grapefruit for
    water.
During last minutes of cooking time add
    grapefruit sections to heat through.
Drain and toss with lemon juice.
Serve in warm bowl; sprinkle lightly with
    cinnamon and pepper.
Serves 6   each: 1 Vegetable Exchange
                     ½ Fruit Exchange

STIR-FRY CABBAGE

½ cup chicken broth
2 tablespoons soy sauce
4 cups thinly sliced cabbage
1 cup sliced celery
1 tablespoon chopped green onion

Heat, in large skillet, chicken broth and soy
    sauce to boiling.
Stir in cabbage, celery and onion.
Cook over high heat, turning vegetables
    frequently with spatula until tender.
Do not overcook.
Serves 4 each: 1 Vegetable Exchange

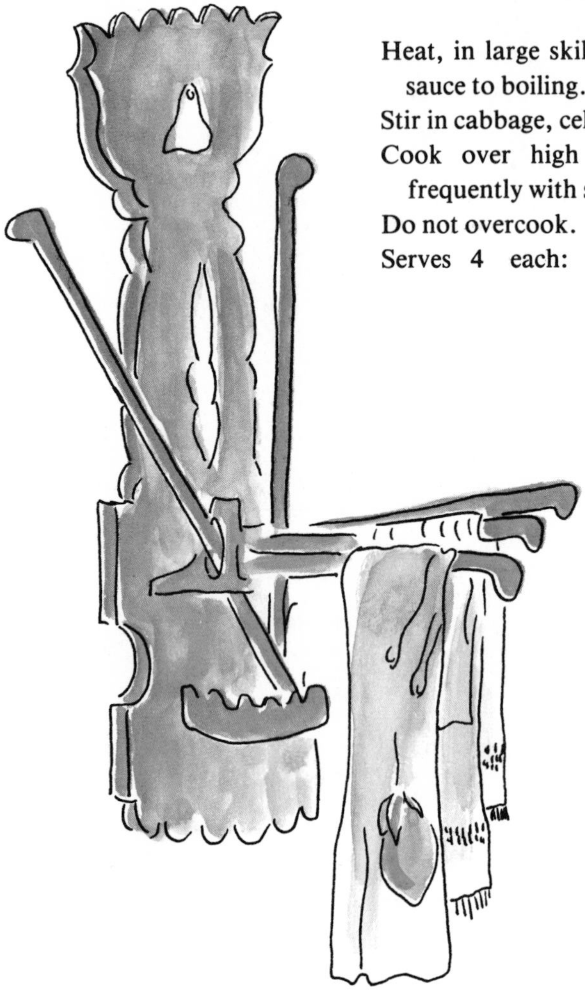

MARINATED CUCUMBERS

1 cucumber, peeled
½ onion, sliced thinly
½ cup vinegar
½ cup water
¼ teaspoon salt
dash fresh ground pepper

Thinly slice cucumber into bowl.
Add onion.
Make marinade from remaining ingredients,
    and pour over vegetables.
Marinate in refrigerator for 1 hour.
Serves 4   each: 1 Vegetable Exchange

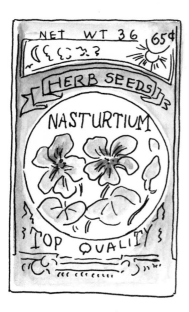

NET WT 36 65¢

HERB SEEDS

NASTURTIUM

TOP QUALITY

JEWEL NASTURTIUM

Tropaelum majus   ANNUAL

USES: The spicy peppery tasting leaves, rich in vitamin C, are an excellent addition to salads and sandwiches. The buds, when pickled, can be substituted for capers.

HEIGHT 12-15" FULL SUN
SOW OUTDOORS IN LATE SPRING
GERMINATES IN 5-10 DAYS

CABBAGE LASAGNA

2 pounds lean ground beef
1 medium onion, chopped
1 green pepper, chopped
1 medium cabbage, shredded
½ teaspoon oregano
1 teaspoon salt
⅛ teaspoon pepper
1 (18-ounce) can tomato paste
8 ounces mozzarella cheese

Saute ground beef, onion and pepper until meat is brown.
Boil cabbage until tender.
Save 2 cups of the liquid and drain off whatever liquid remains.
Combine 2 cups of the reserved cabbage liquid, oregano, salt, pepper and tomato paste and simmer over low heat for 5 minutes.
Add meat, onion and green pepper to tomato mixture into a 9 × 13 inch pan.
Layer cabbage, then remaining tomato mixture.
Top with slices of cheese to cover.
Bake at 400° until cheese is browned, about 30-45 minutes.

Serves 8   each: 4 Meat Exchanges
2 Vegetable Exchanges
½ Bread Exchange
1 Fat Exchange

What father among you, if his son asks
for an egg, will give him a scorpion?

Luke 11:12

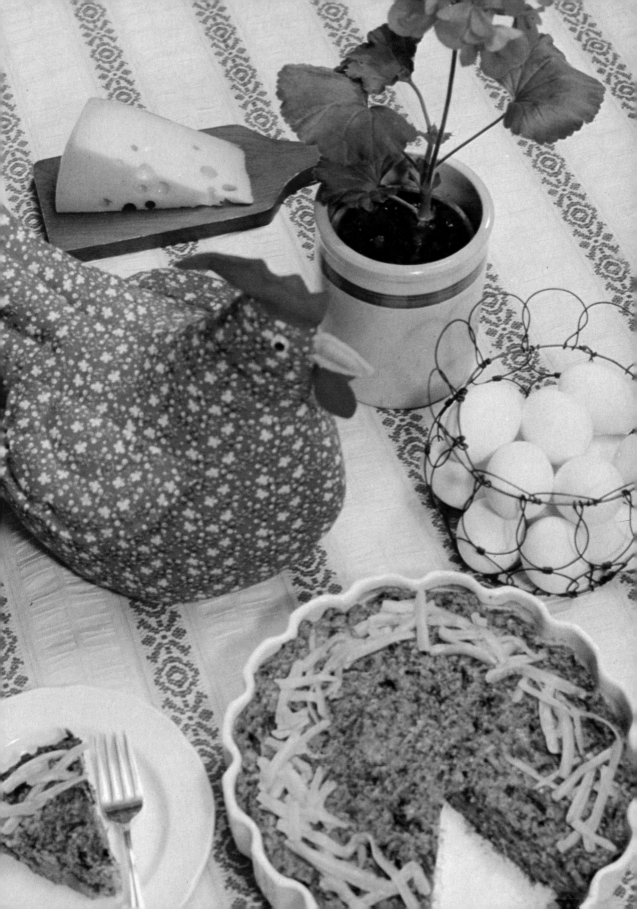

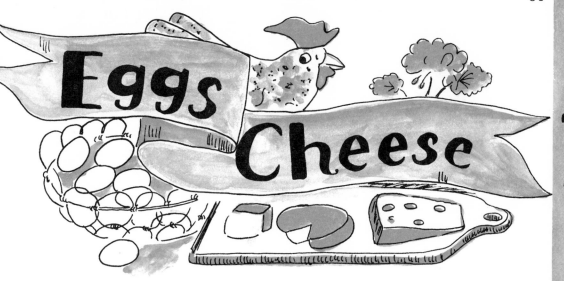

CHEESE-BROCCOLI BAKE

1 package frozen chopped broccoli, cooked
1 egg
½ cup cottage cheese (not creamed)
1 tablespoon minced onion
1 teaspoon beef bouillon powder
Salt and pepper to taste

Cook and drain broccoli.
Put remaining ingredients into a blender.
Blend well.
Mix well with Broccoli.
Put mixture into baking dish and place in pan
  of water.
Bake at 350° for 35-40 minutes.
Serves 4   each: 1 Meat Exchange
                      1 Vegetable Exchange

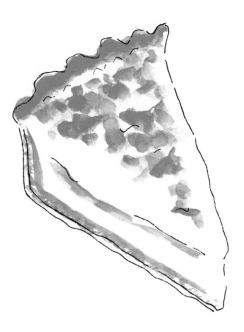

SPINACH QUICHE

1 package frozen chopped spinach
2 cups skim milk
4 eggs, beaten
¼ cup finely chopped onions
4 slices bacon, fried and broken in pieces
½ teaspoon salt
¼ teaspoon paprika
½ teaspoon dry mustard
1 cup shredded cheddar cheese
1 9-inch pie shell
¼ cup more cheese for topping

Cook spinach and drain well.
Mix remaining ingredients and add to spin-
    ach.
Put in unbaked pie shell.
Sprinkle ¼ cup cheese on top.
Bake at 400° for 40 minutes or until set.
Serves 6   each: 2 Meat Exchanges
                    1 Bread Exchange
                    1 Vegetable Exchange
                    2 Fat Exchanges

FRESH MUSHROOM-CHEESE PIE

1 cup shredded Swiss cheese
2 tablespoons flour
2 eggs, beaten
¾ cup skim milk
½ teaspoon dried summer savory
½ teaspoon salt
¼ teaspoon pepper
2 cups sliced mushrooms

Toss shredded cheese with flour in bowl. Add
    eggs, milk and seasonings.
Fold in sliced mushrooms.
Pour into 8-inch pie crust.
Bake at 350° for 1 hour or until brown and
    knife inserted comes clean from center.
Serves 6   each: with crust,
                    2 Meat Exchanges
                    1 Vegetable Exchange
                    1 Bread Exchange
                    1 Fat Exchange

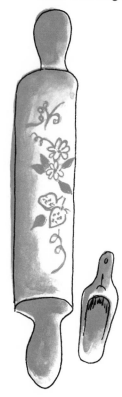

CARROT SOUFFLE

3 cups shredded carrots
⅔ cup brown rice
½ teaspoon salt
1 teaspoon butter
2 cups shredded mild cheddar cheese
1 cup skim milk
2 beaten eggs
1 small chopped onion
¼ teaspoon pepper

In saucepan, combine carrots, rice, salt,
   1 teaspoon butter and 2 cups of water.
Bring to boiling.
Reduce heat and simmer, covered, 40 minutes.
Do not drain.
Stir in 1½ cups of cheese and the milk, eggs,
   onion and pepper.
Turn into 1½-quart casserole.
Bake at 350° for 1 hour.
Top with remaining cheese.
Bake 5 minutes more.
Serves 8   each: 2 Meat Exchanges
                      2 Vegetable Exchanges
                      2 Fat Exchanges

BAKED EGGS

Spray muffin tins with non-stick spray.
Fry bacon slightly, leaving it soft.
Put around inside of muffin tin.
Break egg in center and sprinkle lightly with
   salt and pepper.
Bake at 350° for 15-20 minutes.
Serves 1   1 Meat Exchange
                     1½ Fat Exchanges

egg and cheese

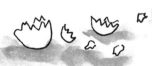
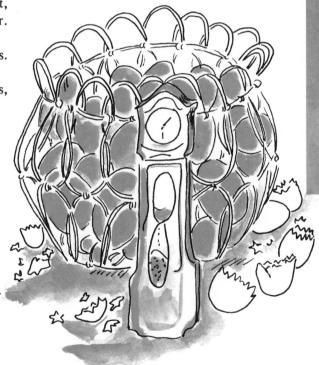

84

ZUCCHINI AND TOMATO OMELET

1 artichoke
1 small sliced zucchini
1 small sliced tomato
4 eggs
½ cup skim milk
Salt and pepper to taste

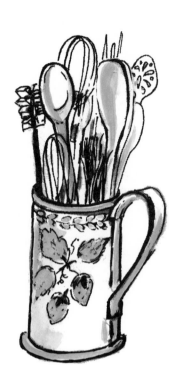

Remove all leaves and chokes from artichoke
and drop the heart with the zucchini in ¼ cup
water; cook until soft.

In blender put eggs, skim milk, salt and pepper and whip until fluffy.

Pour egg mixture into skillet and cook,
scraping edges until only a little uncooked
eggs remain in the center.

Add vegetables and seasonings.

Cover and cook until vegetables are hot.

Turn ½ of omelet and serve.

Serves 2   each:

2 Meat Exchanges   ¼ Milk Exchange
2 Vegetable Exchanges   1 Fat Exchange

CHEESE OMELET

Beat eggs until fluffy.

For each egg, beat in 1 tablespoon water and
a dash of salt and pepper.

Pour into sizzling butter (1 teaspoon per egg)
in skillet over *low* heat.

Cook slowly.

As under-surface becomes set, start lifting it
slightly with spatula to let uncooked portion flow underneath and cook.

Add ½ tablespoon grated cheese for each egg.

As soon as all of the mixture seems set, fold
or roll it.

Serve immediately.

Serves 1 per egg   1 Meat Exchange
                       2 Fat Exchanges

Variation: When the mixture is set, you
may add your favorite vegetable combination or cheese.

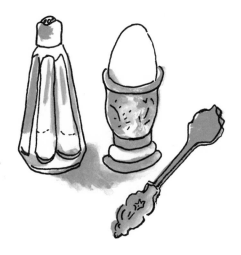

MUSHROOM ASPARAGUS OMELET

1 cup asparagus tips
½ cup chicken bouillon
2 eggs, beaten slightly
1 tablespoon water
½ (4-ounce) can mushroom pieces
Salt and pepper
1 ounce shredded Cheddar cheese

Heat asparagus in chicken bouillon.
Combine eggs, water and mushrooms.
Season with salt and pepper.
Pour into omelet pan.
When eggs are set and surface is still moist, drain hot asparagus.
Place asparagus across the center of the omelet.
Sprinkle with grated cheese.
Fold omelet pan over.
Cook until done.

Serves 2   each: 2 Meat Exchanges
                       1 Vegetable Exchange
                       1 Fat Exchange

SPANISH OMELET

1 egg
1 ounce cheese (Swiss, Edam or your choice)
Salt and pepper to taste
1 tablespoon chopped green pepper
1 tablespoon chopped onion
¼ cup chopped stewed tomatoes

Mix first five ingredients and cook in teflon fry pan as in cheese omelet.
Top with warm stewed tomatoes.

Serves 1   2 Meat Exchanges
                1 Vegetable Exchange
                2 Fat Exchanges

egg and cheese

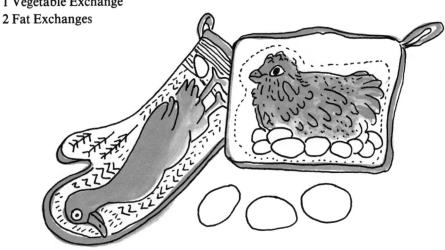

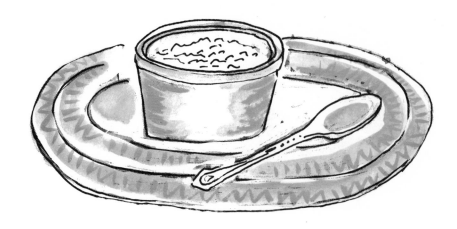

COTTAGE CHEESE ON TOAST

1 slice bread
¼ cup cottage cheese
1 teaspoon cinnamon
Sweetener to taste

Mix cottage cheese, cinnamon and sweetener.
Spread on toast and bake at 375° until hot.
Serves 1   1 Meat Exchange
                     1 Bread Exchange

COTTAGE CHEESE SPREAD

1 slice bacon
¼ cup cottage cheese
1 slice whole wheat toast

Cook crisp and crumble 1 bacon slice per
   serving.
Mix into cottage cheese and spread on toasted
   wheat bread.
Serves 1   1 Meat Exchange
                     1 Bread Exchange
                     1 Fat Exchange

COTTAGE CHEESE FILLED CREPES

½ cup whole wheat flour
½ cup white flour
3 eggs, well beaten
1 tablespoon honey
1 tablespoon oil
½ teaspoon salt
½ teaspoon baking powder
1¼ cups skim milk

Mix all ingredients together.
Blend well.
Pour ¼ cup batter onto hot, lightly buttered
   10-inch griddle.
Spread batter to nearly cover the bottom of
   the pan.
When crepe is bubbly all over, turn.
Place 3 tablespoons cottage cheese in center
   of crepe and continue cooking.
When crepe is browned, fold sides over cot-
   tage cheese and place on plate.
Serves 5   each serving of 2 crepes equals:
                3 Meat Exchanges
                2 Bread Exchanges
Serving Suggestion: Spoon berries or peaches
   over top (optional).

CREPES

3 eggs
6 tablespoons all-purpose flour
½ cup skim milk
2 tablespoons diet margarine, at room temperature
1 teaspoon vanilla

Combine all ingredients in blender and beat until smooth.

Let batter rest 20 minutes. Use a 7-inch pan with a non-stick surface.

Apply cooking spray to pan and heat until moderately hot.

Make 1 crepe at a time.

Rotate pan to spread batter as thin as possible. Cook 30-40 seconds.

Flip pan over onto a clean towel and let crepe fall out.

Apply cooking spray to the skillet for each new crepe.

Makes 12   Each serving of 2 crepes
                    1 Bread Exchange

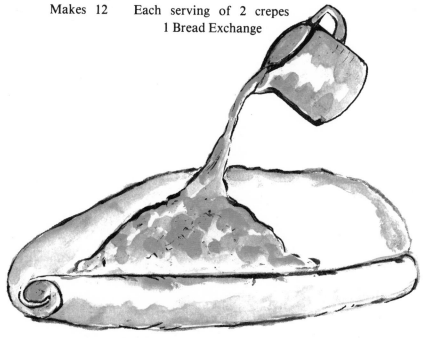

... crepes can be filled with all sorts of vegetables, meats, cheese, and fruits. a great way to turn leftovers into a very special dish~

egg and cheese

GREEN AND RED PEPPER CASEROLE

2 green peppers
2 red peppers (sweet, not hot)
1½ cups sharp cheddar cheese, cubed
6 eggs
½ teaspoon salt
⅛ teaspoon lemon pepper
2 cups skim milk

Remove seeds and stems from peppers and
  cut into ½-inch strips. Steam till ¾ done.
Place in layers in greased casserole, alternat-
  ing with layers of cheese until all are used.
Beat eggs well, add salt and pepper, then milk.
Mix thoroughly and pour over pepper-cheese
  mixture.
Bake in preheated 300° oven for approxi-
  mately 1 hour or until firm in center.
Serves 6   each: 2 Meat Exchanges
                     1 Vegetable Exchange
                     ¼ Milk Exchange
                     2 Fat Exchanges

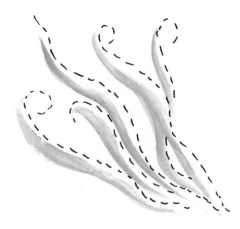

EGGS ON CURRIED RICE

1½ cups brown rice
1 tablespoon butter
2 tablespoons whole wheat flour
2 cups beef bouillon (prepared)
1 teaspoon chopped chives
2 teaspoons curry powder
Salt and pepper to taste
4 eggs
chopped parsley

Cook rice.
Pack cooked rice firmly into greased baking
  dish.
Make four little wells, evenly spaced, in the
  rice.
Melt butter in saucepan, add flour and then
  beef bouillon, stirring constantly.
  stantly.
Cook until thickened.
Add seasonings.
Spoon half of the sauce over the rice into the
  wells.
Break an egg into each well, and gently spoon
  the remaining sauce over the entire surface
  and bake in preheated 350° oven for 25
  minutes or until eggs are firm.
Garnish with chopped parsley.
Serves 4   each: 1 Meat Exchange
                     1 Bread Exchange
                     1 Fat Exchange

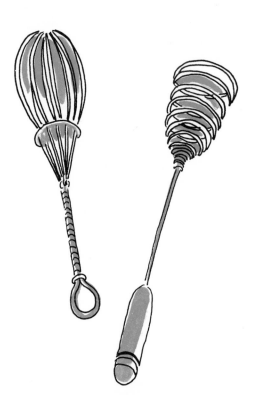

SWISS CHEESE HAWAIIAN

1 small can mushrooms
1 small can crushed unsweetened pineapple
1 packages frozen chopped broccoli
6 ounces Swiss cheese
2 teaspoons mayonnaise
Salt and pepper

In small saucepan cook broccoli; add mushrooms and cook for 1 minute longer.

Place cheese in 6 small slices on top of mixture.

Cover and cook on low heat until cheese is very soft but not liquid; carefully drain excess water. Place mixture in bowl and toss with well-drained pineapple and mayonnaise.

Serves 3   each: 2 Meat Exchanges
                    2 Vegetable Exchanges
                    1 Fruit Exchange
                    2½ Fat Exchanges

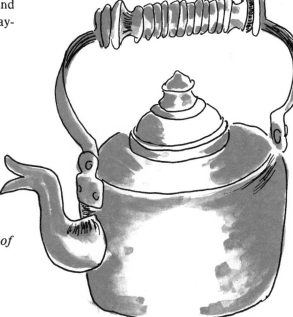

EGGS DELMONICO

1 (10½-ounce) can condensed cream of mushroom soup
¼ cup grated cheese
4 hard-cooked eggs, quartered
2 ounces chopped pimento
Curry powder (optional)

Heat soup over low heat.
Stir in pimento and cheese.
Carefully fold in eggs.
Continue cooking over low heat until cheese is melted.
Serve immediately on dry toast, sprinkle with paprika and garnish with parsley.

Serves 2   each: 3 Meat Exchanges
                    1 Bread Exchange
                    3 Fat Exchanges

egg and cheese

BROCCOLI TIMBALES

1½ pounds broccoli
4 eggs
1½ cups skim milk
½ teaspoon salt
⅛ teaspoon pepper
1 tablespoon chopped parsley
2½ ounces cheddar cheese (grated)

Simmer broccoli in a little water until tender.

Chop broccoli and drain well.

Use 2 cups for this recipe.

In a bowl, combine eggs, milk, salt and pepper and beat with a whisk until well blended.

Add broccoli, cheese and parsley and pour into a greased 1-quart mold or individual molds, filling them approximately ⅔ full.

Place molds in a pan of hot water which reaches half-way up the side of molds.

Bake in preheated 350° oven for 25-45 minutes, depending on the size of the molds. Done when knife inserted in center comes out clean.

Serves 6   each: 1 Meat Exchange
                      1 Vegetable Exchange
                      ½ Milk Exchange
                      ½ Fat Exchange

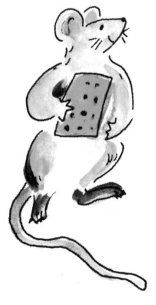

BAKED TOMATOES AND EGGS

4 large tomatoes
1 small onion, minced
1 tablespoon oil
½ cup dry whole grain bread crumbs
1 teaspoon basil
½ teaspoon fennel
Salt and pepper to taste
4 eggs (at room temperature)
½ cup grated Cheddar cheese

Cut out the tops of the tomatoes, then scoop
   out the easy-to-remove pulp.
Saute onion in oil.
Mix ½ cup of pulp with onion, bread crumbs
   and seasonings.
Fill tomato shells approximately ⅓ full with
   crumb mixture.
Break an egg into each tomato and cover with
   grated cheese.
Place each tomato in a greased ramekin and
   bake in preheated 325° oven for 12-15 minutes or until eggs are just set and tomatoes
   are soft but not collapsing.
Be careful not to overcook the eggs.
Serve immediately.

Serves 4   each: 1½ Meat Exchanges
                     1 Bread Exchange
                     1 Vegetable Exchange
                     2 Fat Exchanges

egg and cheese

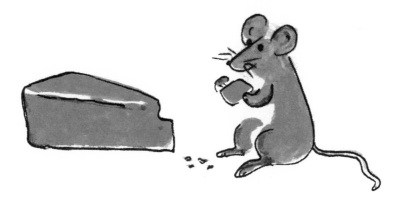

"But of all clean fowls ye may eat."

Deuteronomy 14:20

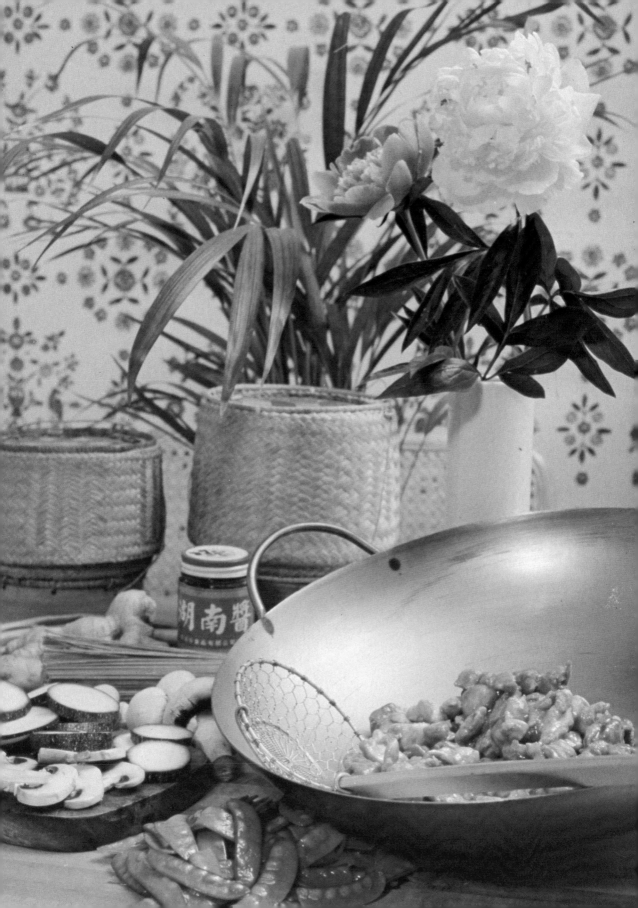

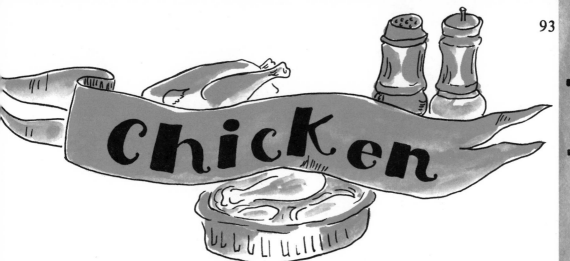

CHICKEN AND VEGETABLE
STIR-FRY

3 large whole chicken breasts (about 2½
  pounds)
1 tablespoon cornstarch
3 tablespoons soy sauce
2 tablespoons dry sherry
1 teaspoon sugar
1 teaspoon ground ginger
¼ - ½ teaspoon crushed red pepper
salt
3 medium zucchini
1 (6-ounce) package frozen Chinese pea pods
  (snow peas)
1 pound small mushrooms
½ cup salad oil

Remove bones from chicken breasts; cut chicken into 1½-inch chunks.

In medium bowl, mix chicken, cornstarch, soy sauce, sherry, sugar, ginger, crushed red pepper and 2½ teaspoons salt.

Cut zucchini into bite-size pieces.

Thaw frozen pea pods with running hot water; pat dry with paper towels.

Quickly rinse mushrooms with running cold water; pat dry with paper towels.

Heat oil in 8-quart Dutch oven or wok over medium-high heat; cook zucchini and mushrooms with ½ teaspoon salt until zucchini is tender-crisp, stirring constantly

with slotted spoon (about 5 minutes).

Spoon zucchini mix onto platter, leaving oil in Dutch oven.

In remaining oil, cook chicken mix until chicken is tender, stirring frequently (about 10 minutes).

Add snow peas and zucchini mix; toss gently to mix well; heat through.

Serve immediately.

Accompany with hot, fluffy rice (optional).

Serves 6   each: 4 Meat Exchanges
                  1 Vegetable Exchange
                  2 Fat Exchanges

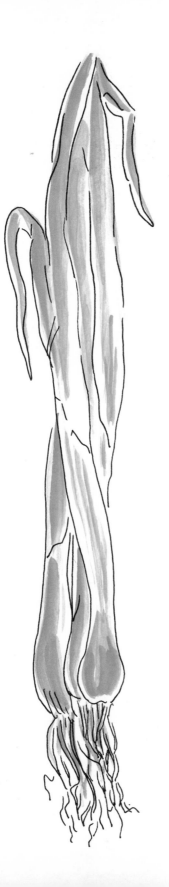

CHICKEN CHOW MEIN
(Cantonese Style)

1 (10-ounce) package frozen mixed Chinese-
style vegetables in sauce
2 teaspoons cornstarch
1 tablespoon soy sauce
2 whole chicken breasts, skinned, boned and
cut into thin strips
(or 2 cups slivered cooked chicken)
3 teaspoons vegetable oil
¼ cup chopped green onion
1 can condensed chicken broth
2 tablespoons dry sherry
1½ cups very fine noodles
1 (8-ounce) package frozen, cooked, shelled
and deveined shrimp
2 cups finely shredded romaine lettuce
(or 1 cup bean sprouts)

Remove vegetables from package; let thaw in
large bowl until vegetables can be separated
with a fork.
Combine cornstarch and soy sauce with
chicken in medium-size bowl.
Heat oil in wok or large skillet until very hot.
Add chicken mixture and stir-fry until chicken
turns white and the pieces separate.
(If using cooked chicken, stir-fry 30 seconds
until hot.)
With a slotted spoon, remove chicken to a
plate.
Add 1 more teaspoon of oil if necessary.
Stir in green onions.
Add broth and sherry; cover; bring to
boiling.
Stir in noodles and let boil about one minute.
Stir in partially thawed vegetables and cook
uncovered for 1 minute.
Add chicken and the frozen shrimp.
Stir-fry until noodles are tender and chicken
and shrimp are heated through.
Stir in lettuce or bean sprouts; serve immedi-
ately.
Serves 6   each: 3 Meat Exchanges
1 Vegetable Exchange
1 Bread Exchange
Sprinkle with chow mein noodles (optional).

CHICKEN GOULASH

1 small fryer, cut up, skin removed
⅓ cup olive oil
½ cup chopped onions
3 cups chopped stewed tomatoes
¼ cup dry white wine
½ teaspoon salt
dash of pepper
½ bay leaf
dash of thyme
¼ teaspoon marjoram

Brown chicken in oil.
Add remaining ingredients.
Cover and simmer 1-1½ hours until meat comes off bones.
Cool and bone chicken.
Place chicken pieces in sauce and reheat.
Serve over rice or noodles (optional).
Serves 6   each: 4 Meat Exchanges
1 Vegetable Exchange
1 Fat Exchange

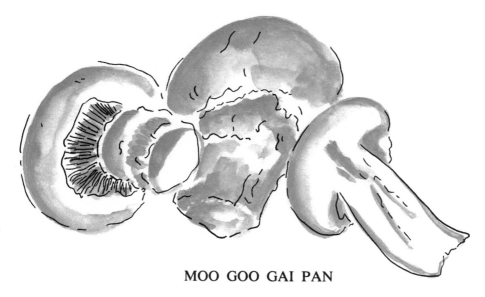

MOO GOO GAI PAN

2 cups cooked chicken, slivered
1 teaspoon cornstarch
3 teaspoons dry sherry
2 teaspoons salt
4 tablespoons oil
1 clove garlic, peeled
½ cup bamboo shoots, diced
½ cup water chestnuts, sliced
3 cups broccoli, diced
2 cups fresh mushrooms, sliced, or 4-oz. can

Have all vegetables ready to use.
Mix chicken with sherry, cornstarch and salt.
Heat oil in wok or frying pan.
Press garlic into hot oil or mince garlic into oil and fry until golden.
Immediately add chicken.
Stir-fry about 2 minutes or until meat turns white.
Add broccoli and mushrooms.
Stir-fry 2 minutes more.
Add water chestnuts and bamboo shoots and stir-fry another couple of minutes.

Serves 4   each: 4 Meat Exchanges
2 Vegetable Exchanges
1 Fat Exchange
Serve immediately, over rice if desired (optional).

chicken

BAKED MARINATED CHICKEN

2½-pound broiler-fryer, cut up and skinned
2 tablespoons lemon juice
2 tablespoons soy sauce
1 teaspoon dry mustard
2 teaspoons salad oil

Combine above ingredients in large bowl and
 dip chicken pieces in it to coat well.
Marinate in refrigerator at least 4 hours or
 overnight, turning occasionally.
Bake in shallow pan, flesh side down.
Cover with marinade.
Bake at 400° for 20 minutes, then turn and
 bake 30 minutes longer, basting occasionally with juices.

Serves 6   each: 4 Meat Exchanges
                     1 Fat Exchange

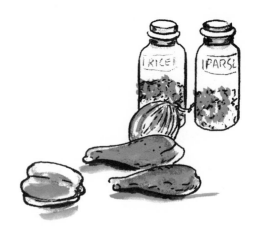

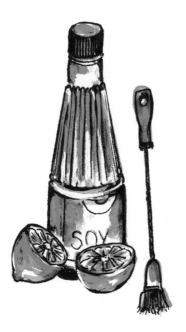

CHICKEN AND RICE BAKE

1 (10¾-ounce) can cream of mushroom soup
¾ cup long grain rice
½ cup skim milk
2 tablespoons minced celery
½ teaspoon salt
⅛ teaspoon pepper
3 pounds chicken parts
paprika

In 13x9-inch baking pan stir first six ingredi-
 ents.
Sprinkle chicken with paprika.
Arrange chicken pieces over mixture.
Cover tightly with foil.
Bake at 375° for 45 minutes.
Remove foil; bake 20 minutes longer or until
 tender.

Serves 8   each: 4 Meat Exchanges
                     1 Bread Exchange
                     ½ Milk Exchange

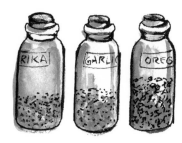

SLIM-JIM BAKED CHICKEN

1 teaspoon fresh grated lemon peel
1 teaspoon paprika
½ teaspoon garlic salt
½ teaspoon oregano
1 whole chicken (cut up and skinned)
1 tablespoon fresh squeezed lemon juice

Combine lemon peel, paprika, garlic salt and
  oregano.
Rub well into all sides of chicken.
Arrange chicken flesh-side down on rack in
  shallow baking pan.
Lay foil over top of chicken.
Bake at 400° for 40 minutes.
Remove foil; turn chicken and sprinkle
  with lemon juice.
Continue baking uncovered for 20 minutes
  or until tender.
Garnish with parsley if desired.
Serves 4   each: 4 Meat Exchanges

BARBECUE-STYLE CHICKEN

3 pounds chicken pieces
½ cup whole wheat flour
½ teaspoon paprika
¼ cup vegetable oil
½ cup sliced onions
1 medium green pepper in strips
2 cups tomato juice
3 tablespoons apple cider vinegar

Shake chicken in a bag containing flour and
  paprika.
In a large skillet brown chicken in hot oil.
Cover and cook over low heat 30-40 minutes.
Remove chicken from skillet.
Cook onions and green pepper until soft and
  light brown.
Add tomato juice and vinegar.
Cover and simmer 5 minutes.
Add chicken to sauce.
Cook about 20 minutes.
Turn chicken twice and baste.
Serves 6   each: 4 Meat Exchanges
                      1 Bread Exchange
                      ½ Vegetable Exchange
                      1 Fat Exchange

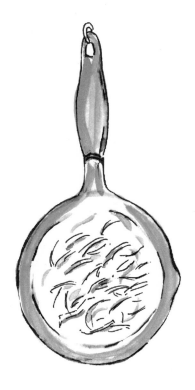

chicken

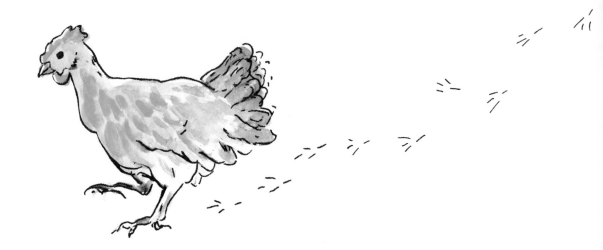

POT O' GOLD CHICKEN

1/3 cup flour
2 teaspoons salt
1/8 teaspoon pepper
1 cut-up chicken
3 tablespoons salad oil
1 cup juice (from juice-packed cling peaches, drained)
1/2 teaspoon dry mustard
1/4 cup chopped onion
1/2 cup orange juice
1 (1 pound 13-ounce) can cling peaches
1 (10-ounce) package frozen peas

Combine flour, salt and pepper in paper bag.
Shake chicken pieces in flour mixture until coated.
Reserve flour mixture.
Brown chicken in oil in large skillet.
Blend peach juice with flour mixture and mustard; add onion and orange juice.
Cook until thick, stirring constantly.
Pour over chicken; cover and simmer for 20 minutes.
Add peach slices and peas.
Cover and simmer 10 minutes longer.
Do not overcook.

Serves 6   each: 4 Meat Exchanges
2 Fruit Exchanges
1 Bread Exchange
1 Fat Exchange

CHICK IN A CROCK-POT

1 chicken, cut in quarters
salt and pepper
1 onion, sliced thin in rings
¼ teaspoon basil or chicken seasoning

Layer in crock-pot and cook on low for 7-8
   hours.
Skim fat off broth before serving.
Serves 4   each: 4 Meat Exchanges
Serve with rice (optional).

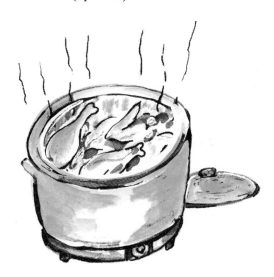

CHICKEN CACCIATORE

3 pounds chicken parts
¼ cup flour
½ teaspoon salt
dash of pepper
⅛ cup salad oil
3 medium onions, chopped
1 green pepper, cut in strips
1 (4-ounce) can mushrooms, drained
1 clove garlic minced (optional)
1 cup V-8 juice
½ teaspoon oregano

Combine flour, salt and pepper.
Dust chicken with flour.
Brown chicken in salad oil in large skillet;
   remove chicken.
Brown onions and green pepper in same pan.
Add mushrooms and garlic.
Blend in remaining ingredients.
Add chicken and cover.
Simmer about 30 minutes or until chicken is
   tender.
Stir occasionally.
Serves 8   each: 4 Meat Exchanges
                     ½ Bread Exchange
                     1 Vegetable Exchange
Serve with spaghetti (optional).

chicken

ORANGE BAKED CHICKEN

3 large chicken breasts, split and skinned
¼ cup orange juice
1 teaspoon grated orange peel
2 tablespoons soy sauce
½ teaspoon ground cinnamon, ginger or
* curry powder*
pepper

Wash and dry chicken breasts; place in
13x9x2-inch baking dish.

Combine other ingredients; pour over
chicken.

Cover; refrigerate about 2 hours, occasionally spooning orange mixture over chicken.

Bake at 350° for 45-60 minutes. Or, for
barbequed chicken, drain marinade,
reserving liquid.

Broil chicken until crisp and brown; turn to
brown on second side.

Meanwhile, cook marinade to serve hot over
broiled chicken.

Serves 6   each: 4 Meat Exchanges

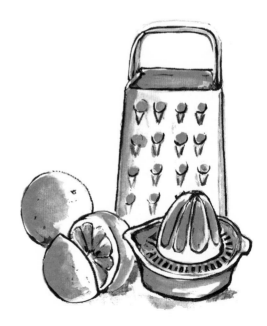

CHICKEN LIVERS ON TOAST

⅓ cup flour
1 pound chicken livers
¼ cup butter
Sauce:
¼ cup chopped onion
¼ cup chopped green pepper
¼ cup flour
½ teaspoon salt
½ teaspoon thyme
½ teaspoon rosemary
⅛ teaspoon pepper
1 cup skim milk
1 cup chicken broth
1 cup sliced mushrooms
6 slices white bread, toasted and cut in half
    diagonally.

Dredge chicken livers in flour.
Saute in butter until golden brown and fully
    cooked, about 15 minutes.
Remove from pan and keep hot.
Reserve remaining butter for sauce.
For sauce:
    Saute onion and green pepper in left-
    over butter until tender (about 5
    minutes).
    Add flour and seasonings and stir until
    smooth.
    Remove from heat.
    Stir in milk and broth.
    Heat to boiling, then stir for 1 minute.
    Stir in mushrooms.
To serve:
    Place 2 toast triangles on each plate.
    Divide chicken livers evenly on toast,
    then top with sauce.
Serves 6   each: 2 Meat Exchanges
                   2 Bread Exchanges
                   1 Fat Exchange

POLYNESIAN CHICKEN LIVERS

4 cups boiling water
6 ounces chicken livers
2 green peppers, chopped
1 medium onion, chopped
1 cup bean sprouts
½ cup chicken bouillon (prepared)
1 teaspoon salt
¼ teaspoon ginger
pepper to taste
¼ cup mushrooms, sliced
1 cup pineapple chunks
2 tablespoons cider vinegar
2 tablespoons corn starch, dissolved in:
4 tablespoons pineapple juice

In a large skillet, boil livers in water for 1
    minute; discard liquid.
Add peppers, bean sprouts, onion, salt,
    ginger, pepper, mushrooms and bouillon.
Cook, covered, for 10 minutes.
Add pineapple.
Stir in vinegar and dissolved cornstarch.
Simmer and stir until mixture thickens.
Serves 2   each: 3 Meat Exchanges
                      ½ Bread Exchange
                      2 Vegetable Exchanges
                      1 Fruit Exchange
Serve over buttered rice (optional)

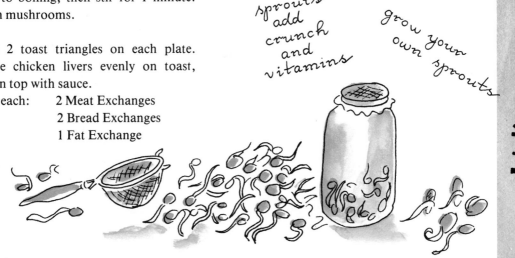

sprouts add crunch and vitamins

grow your own sprouts

chicken

CHICKEN CORDON BLEU

3 large chicken breasts, boned, skinned and
  cut lengthwise
6 thin slices of boiled ham
6 oz. natural Swiss cheese, cut in 6 sticks
¼ cup flour
2 tablespoons diet margarine
1 teaspoon chicken-flavored gravy base
1 (3-ounce) can sliced mushrooms, drained
  (½ cup)
⅓ cup Sauterne wine
2 tablespoons flour
toasted sliced almonds

Roll chicken pieces, boned side up, on cutting
  board.
Working from center out, pound chicken
  with a wooden mallet to make cutlets
  ¼-inch thick.
Sprinkle with salt.
Place a ham slice and a cheese stick on each
  cutlet.
Tuck in sides of each and roll up as for a jelly
  roll.
Skewer or tie securely.
Coat rolls with the ¼ cup flour, brown in
  margarine, and remove to 11x7x1½-inch
  baking pan
In the same skillet, combine ½ cup water, the
  gravy base, mushrooms and wine.
Heat, stirring in the crispy bits from the
  skillet.
Pour mixture over chicken in the baking pan.
Cover and bake at 350° for 1¼ hours, or
  until tender.
Transfer to serving platter.
Pour juices over chicken and garnish with
  toasted sliced almonds.
Serves 6   each: 4 Meat Exchanges
                   ½ Bread Exchange
                   2 Fat Exchanges

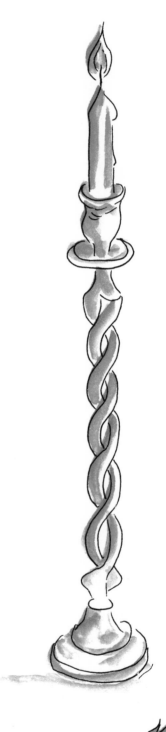

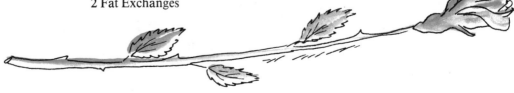

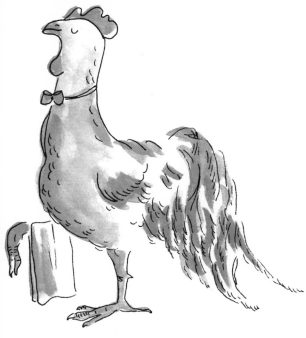

CHICKEN CREPES ELEGANTE

1 recipe crepes (page 87)
¼ chopped onion
¼ cup water
1 cup skim milk
¼ cup all-purpose flour
¼ teaspoon salt
1½ cups shredded cheese
1 (4-ounce) can sliced mushrooms, drained
2 cups finely diced cooked chicken
1 (10-ounce) package frozen, chopped broccoli, cooked and drained

Mushroom sauce:
In saucepan, combine onion and water.
Cook, covered, five minutes, but do not drain.
Blend together milk, flour and salt; add to onion.
Cook and stir until bubbly.
Add shredded cheese, stirring until melted.
Reserve ½ cup of the sauce.
Add mushrooms to remaining sauce; cover and set aside.

Filling:
Combine chicken, broccoli and the ½ cup of reserved sauce.
Spoon about ¼ cup filling on unbrowned side of each crepe; roll up.
Arrange crepes, seam side up, in 13x9x2-inch baking dish.
Bake in 350° oven for 20 minutes.
Heat mushroom sauce; serve over crepes.
Serves 6   each serving of 2 crepes is:
    3 Meat Exchanges
    1 Bread Exchange
    1 Vegetable Exchange
    ½ Milk Exchange
    1 Fat Exchange

CURRIED CHICKEN

8 ounces boneless chicken, cubed
2 tablespoons minced onion
1 teaspoon curry powder
¾ cup chicken bouillon (prepared)
2 tablespoons chopped celery
1 cup tomato juice, cooked down to half
½ apple, chopped
2 carrots, chopped
½ teaspoon lemon juice
salt to taste

Place chicken and onion in non-stick skillet.
Cook over low heat until lightly browned.
Sprinkle curry powder over chicken and stir with wooden spoon.
Add bouillon and celery.
Simmer 10 minutes.
Add tomato juice, carrots, apple and lemon juice.
Simmer until carrots are tender, about 15 minutes.
Season to taste.
Serves 2   each: 3 Meat Exchanges
    ½ Bread Exchange
    1 Vegetable Exchange
Serve over rice (optional).

When they got out on land, they saw a charcoal fire there, with fish lying on it, and bread.

John 21:9

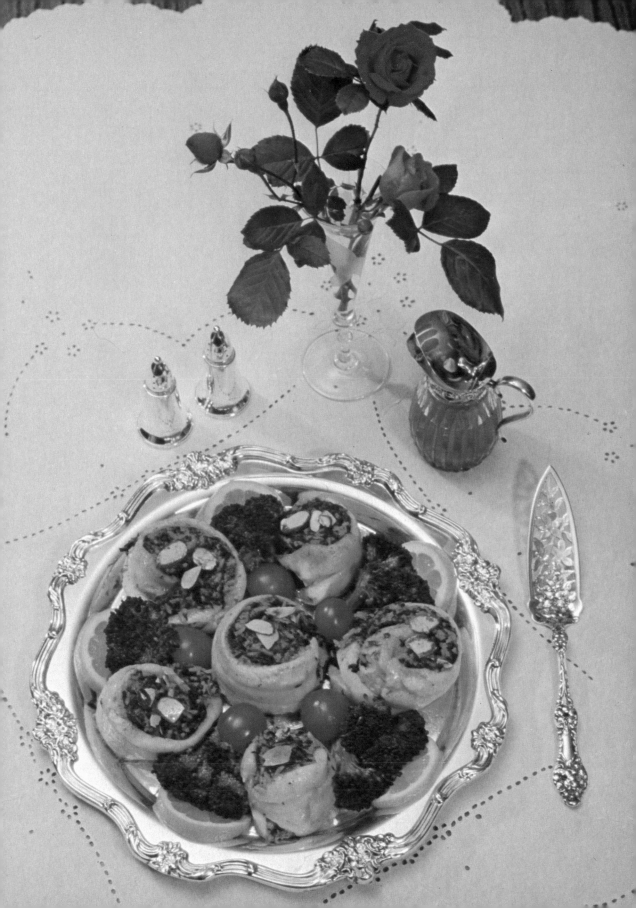

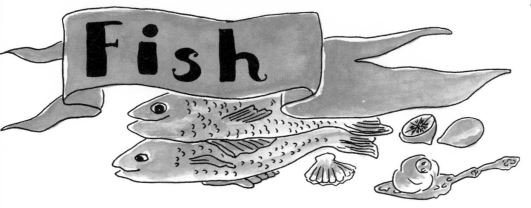

FISH ROLL-UPS

⅓ cup butter or margarine
⅓ cup lemon juice
2 teaspoons chicken bouillon
⅛ teaspoon pepper sauce
2 (10-ounce) packages frozen broccoli, thawed
1 cup cooked rice
1 cup shredded sharp cheddar cheese
10 fish fillets (2 pounds), thawed
paprika

Heat together melted butter, lemon juice, bouillon and pepper sauce until bouillon dissolves.

Combine broccoli, rice, cheese and ¼ cup lemon butter sauce; mix well.

Divide broccoli mixture equally among fillets.

Roll up and place seam down in shallow baking dish.

Pour remaining sauce over roll-ups.

Bake in a preheated 375° oven for 25 minutes or until fish flakes with fork.

Sprinkle with paprika.

Serves 10   each: 4 Meat Exchanges
                     ½ Bread Exchange
                     1 Vegetable Exchange
                     1 Fat Exchange

FRESH FISH

2 pounds fresh blue or white fish

Place in pan lined with foil.
Cover with salt, pepper and tomato slices.
Add parsley, oregano, lemon juice and 2 tea-
 spoons olive oil.
Cover and bake at 350° for 45 minutes.
Serves 8   each: 4 Meat Exchanges
                    ½ Vegetable Exchange

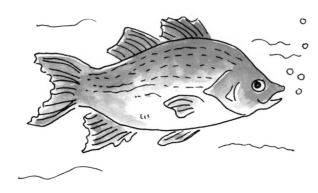

BAKED TURBOT
IN TOMATO JUICE

1 pound turbot fillets
⅓ cup skim milk powder
salt, pepper, thyme to taste
½ cup tomato juice

Roll turbot fillets in milk powder.
Place turbot in baking dish.
Sprinkle with seasonings.
Spoon tomato juice over fish.
Bake at 350° for 45-60 minutes.
Serves 4   each: 4 Meat Exchanges
                    ½ Milk Exchange

LEMON WHITEFISH BAKE

1 ½ pounds whitefish, thawed
3 tablespoons lemon juice
1 teaspoon salt
½ teaspoon paprika
½ cup chopped onion
2 tablespoons butter or margarine

Divide the whitefish into 6 fillets.
In a shallow dish combine juice, salt and
  paprika.
Add whitefish and marinate for 1 hour, turn-
  ing after 30 minutes.
Saute onion in melted butter until tender but
  not brown.
Place fish in greased baking dish.
Top with 6 green pepper strips.
Sprinkle with sauteed onion.
Bake at 450° about 10 minutes or until fish
  flakes easily.
Do not overbake.
Serves 6 each: 4 Meat Exchanges
                    1 Fat Exchange

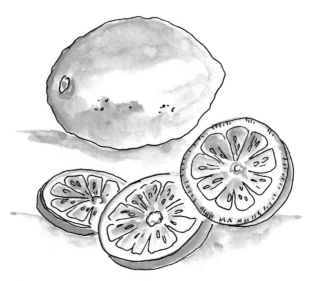

LEMON BAKED FISH FILLETS

1 pound fish fillets
¼ cup water
2 tablespoons lemon juice or dry white wine
4 lemon slices

Arrange fish fillets in a small baking dish.
Sprinkle with seasoned salt and pepper; top
  with lemon slices.
Add the water and lemon juice or white wine.
Cover and bake at 400° for about 15 minutes
  just until fish flakes with a fork.
Garnish with lemon wedges.
Serves 4 each: 4 Meat Exchanges
Place fish on a platter with cooked carrots
and asparagus sprinkled with fresh chopped
  parsley (optional).

108

OVEN POACHED HADDOCK

2 pounds haddock fillets
3 tomatoes, sliced
juice of 1 lemon
1 teaspoon chopped parsley
⅛ teaspoon thyme
½ teaspoon sugar
1 small onion, minced
salt and pepper to taste
2 tablespoons butter

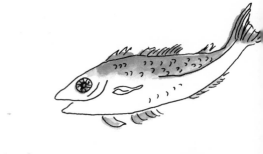

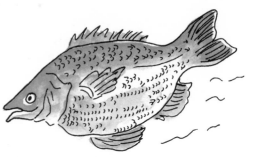

Mix all but fish and tomatoes.
Marinate the haddock in the mixture for 3-4
  hours in the refrigerator.
Place the fish in a baking dish.
Pour marinade over it.
Cover with tomato slices.
Bake at 350° for 40 minutes.
Serves 8   each: 4 Meat Exchanges

PINEAPPLE-PERCH FILLETS

1 pound fresh or frozen perch fillets, thawed
½ cup pineapple juice
1 tablespoon lime juice
4 lime slices
2 teaspoons Worcestershire sauce
½ teaspoon salt
dash of pepper

Cut fillets into 4 portions.
Place in shallow dish.
Combine remaining ingredients, except lime
  slices

Pour over fish and marinate fish in refriger-
  ator 1 hour, turning once.
Drain; reserve marinade.
Place fillets on greased rack of broiler pan
Broil 4 inches from heat until fish flakes
  easily when tested with a fork (about 10
  minutes).
Brush occasionally with marinade.
Heat remaining marinade and spoon over fish
  before serving.
Trim with lime twists.
Serves 4   each: 3 Meat Exchanges
                   ½ Fruit Exchange

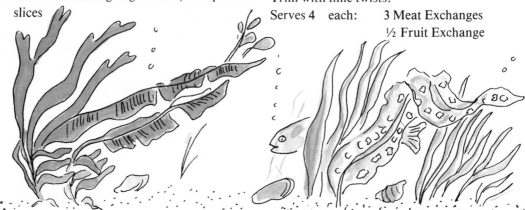

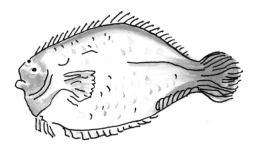

fish

FLOUNDER CONTINENTAL

1 pound fresh or frozen flounder, thawed
1 cup sliced fresh mushrooms
¼ cup chopped onions
1 tablespoon butter or margarine
3 tablespoons flour
½ teaspoon instant chicken bouillon granules
¼ teaspoon seasoned salt
1 cup skim milk
1 teaspoon lemon juice
1 tablespoon snipped parsley

for variety~ ginger and scallions with fish

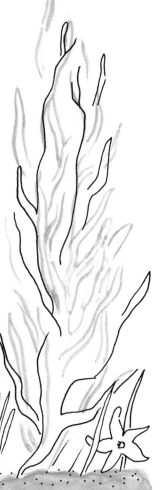

In saucepan cook mushrooms and onion in
  butter till tender but not brown.
Stir in flour, bouillon and seasoned salt.
Stir in milk all at once; cook and stir till mix-
  ture is thick and bubbly.
Place fish in single layer in 11x7½x1½-inch
  baking pan.
Sprinkle lightly with salt and drizzle with
  lemon juice.
Spoon mushroom mixture atop fish.
Cover and bake at 325° till fish flakes easily
  (about 25 minutes).
Transfer to serving platter and sprinkle with
  snipped parsley.
Serves 4   each: 4 Meat Exchanges
                     1 Vegetable Exchange
                     ¼ Milk Exchange

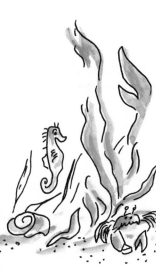

BAKED FISH

4 ounces fish (cod, flounder, ocean perch)
2 tablespoons water
2 teaspoons butter
3 tablespoons bread crumbs
1 teaspoon lemon juice, pepper, thyme (optional)
paprika

Place fish in shallow baking pan.

Melt together butter, bread crumbs, lemon juice, pepper, and thyme.

Spread on top of fish; add dash of paprika.

Bake uncovered at 350° about 20-30 minutes or until fish flakes when touched with fork.

Serves 1   4 Meat Exchanges
                 1 Bread Exchange
                 1 Fat Exchange

FISH CHOWDER

1 medium-size onion, minced
½ cup diced celery
½ cup diced carrot
3 tablespoons butter or margarine
3 medium-size potatoes, peeled
1 cup prepared chicken bouillon
½ cup skim milk powder
1 cup water
1 pound fish fillet
1 bay leaf
salt and pepper to taste
1-2 tablespoons cider vinegar
snipped chives

Using a large saucepan, saute onion, celery and carrot in butter till onions are translucent.

Cube or grate potatoes and add to sauteed vegetables.

Stir in bouillon and bring to a boil.

Simmer until vegetables are almost done.

Reconstitute milk with cup of water and add to soup.

Add fish and bay leaf and simmer for 20-30 minutes or until fish is tender.

Flake fish into bite-size pieces.

Season to taste with salt, pepper and vinegar.

Garnish with snipped chives and serve.

Serves 4 each: 4 Meat Exchanges
                      1 Bread Exchange
                      1 Vegetable Exchange
                      ½ Milk Exchange
                      1 Fat Exchange

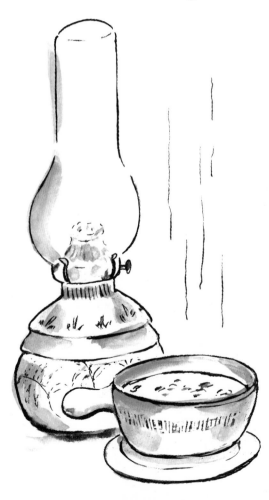

BAKED SALMON LOAF

1 pound can of salmon
1 cup shredded American cheese
1 cup cracker or dry bread crumbs
1 tablespoon grated onion
1 teaspoon lemon juice
½ teaspoon dill weed
½ teaspoon celery salt
¼ teaspoon salt
pepper
1 egg, beaten
⅔ cup skim milk
2 tablespoons melted butter

Flake salmon, add remaining ingredients and
   mix well.
Place in a greased 1-quart loaf pan.
Bake at 350° for 35-40 minutes or until lightly
   browned.
Serves 6   each: 4 Meat Exchanges
                   ½ Bread Exchange
                   ½ Fat Exchange

SALMON CROQUETTES

1 (3-ounce) can salmon, drained and flaked
1 teaspoon dehydrated onion flakes
4 tablespoons finely chopped celery
mustard, enough to moisten

Mix all ingredients and make into patties.
Place on foil.
Bake 20 minutes in 350° oven.
Broil until lightly browned.
Serves 1   2 Meat Exchanges

fish

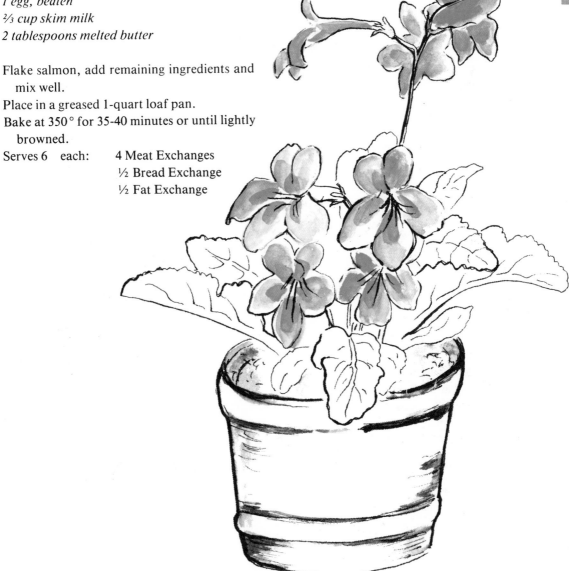

TUNA MELT

3 ounces water-packed tuna fish
1 teaspoon lemon juice
2 pineapple rings (packed in own juice)
1 ounce cheese
1 English muffin

Mash tuna and moisten with lemon juice.
Split muffin and toast lightly.
Place one pineapple ring on each, fill with
  tuna.
Cover with strips of cheese and broil.
Chopped celery or onion or crushed pine-
  apple may be added with the tuna.
Serves 2   each: 2 Meat Exchanges
                   1 Bread Exchange
                   1 Fruit Exchange
                   1 Fat Exchange

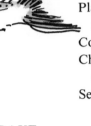

SHRIMP AND TUNA BAKE

⅔ cup long grain rice
1 (9-ounce) package frozen green beans
1 (10½-ounce) can cream of celery soup
½ cup skim milk
2 tablespoons chopped canned pimento
¼ teaspoon dried thyme, crushed
dash cayenne
1 (6½-ounce) can tuna, drained and broken
  into chunks
1 (4½-ounce) can shrimp, drained

Cook rice according to package directions.
Cook green beans according to package
  directions.
Drain; set aside.
Combine next 5 ingredients; stir until
  smooth.
Stir half of sauce mixture into rice, fold in
  tuna, turn into 1½-quart casserole.
Spread green beans over rice and top with
  shrimp.
Pour remaining sauce over all.
Bake covered at 325° until heated through,
  25-30 minutes.
Serves 4   each: 2 Meat Exchanges
                   1 Bread Exchange
                   ½ Vegetable Exchange

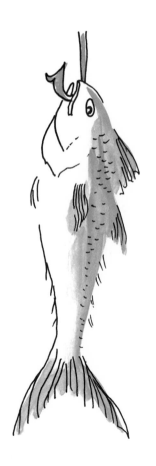

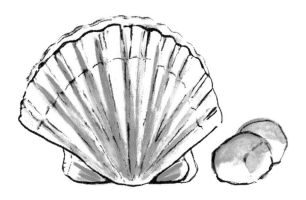

BROILED SCALLOPS

1 tablespoon salad oil
1 small garlic clove, crushed
¾ teaspoon salt
2 tablespoons chopped parsley
1 pound sea scallops, cut into bite-size pieces
1 tablespoon butter, melted
½ cup fresh bread crumbs
paprika

In medium bowl mix oil, garlic, salt and parsley.

Add scallops and stir; marinate for 1 hour in refrigerator.

Preheat broiler.

Toss melted butter with bread crumbs.

Spoon scallops and marinade into a shallow flame-proof dish or 4 individual ramekins.

Place 2 inches from broiler; then broil 3 minutes.

Turn scallops, sprinkle with bread crumbs and paprika and broil 3 minutes more.

Serves 4   each: 3 Meat Exchanges
                     ½ Bread Exchange
                     ½ Fat Exchange

STIR-FRIED WHITEFISH

1½ pounds white fish fillets

½ tablespoon white wine
½ teaspoon salt

1 egg white
½ tablespoon cornstarch

2 tablespoons oil

*1 tablespoon minced scallions, including the
    green part*
1 tablespoon minced fresh ginger
1½ tablespoons white wine

½ teaspoon salt
2 teaspoons sugar
2 teaspoons cornstarch
½ cup chicken stock

Slice the fillets thinly and marinate in first
    mixture for 20 minutes. Combine ingredi-
    ents in second mixture and add to the fish.
Put oil in hot frying pan.
Put ingredients for third mixture in fry pan;
    stir-fry for 1 minute.
Add ingredients for fourth mixture and stir-
    fry until bubbling.
Add the fish mixture; stir-fry for 5 minutes.
Serves 6   each: 4 Meat Exchanges
                               1 Fat Exchange

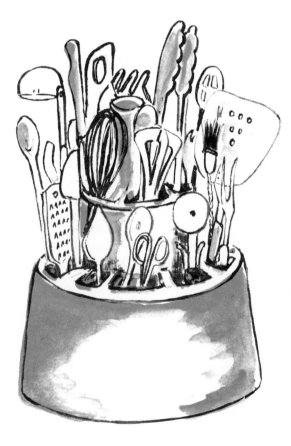

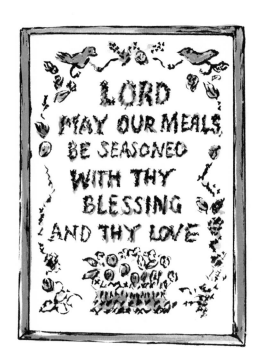

fish

SPICY RED SNAPPER

2½-3 pounds red snapper
2 quarts water
⅓ cup finely-shredded fresh ginger*
½ cup shredded white part of scallions
½ cup shredded green part of scallions
½ cup peanut, vegetable or corn oil
¼ cup thinly shredded, seeded fresh red or
*   green sweet or hot peppers*
1 cup chicken broth
¼ teaspoon monosodium glutamate
*   (optional)*
salt to taste
1 tablespoon cornstarch
¼ cup cold water

* available in Chinese markets

Place the fish in a plate and fit the plate inside
    the top of a steamer. Fit the top over the
    bottom and steam the fish over boiling
    water for exactly 15 minutes.
Remove the fish and pour off the liquid that
    has accumulated around it. Scatter the
    ginger and half the scallions and peppers
    over the fish.
Heat the oil in a small skillet; when it is
    almost piping hot, but not smoking, pour
    it over the fish.
Bring the broth to a boil and add the mono-
    sodium glutamate and salt. Blend the corn-
    starch and the water and stir into the sauce.
    When thickened, pour the sauce over the
    fish. Scatter the remaining scallions and
    peppers over the fish and serve hot.
Serves 8   each: 4 Meat Exchanges
                    1 Vegetable Exchange

She rises while it is yet night and provides meat for her household and tasks for her maidens.

Proverbs 31:15

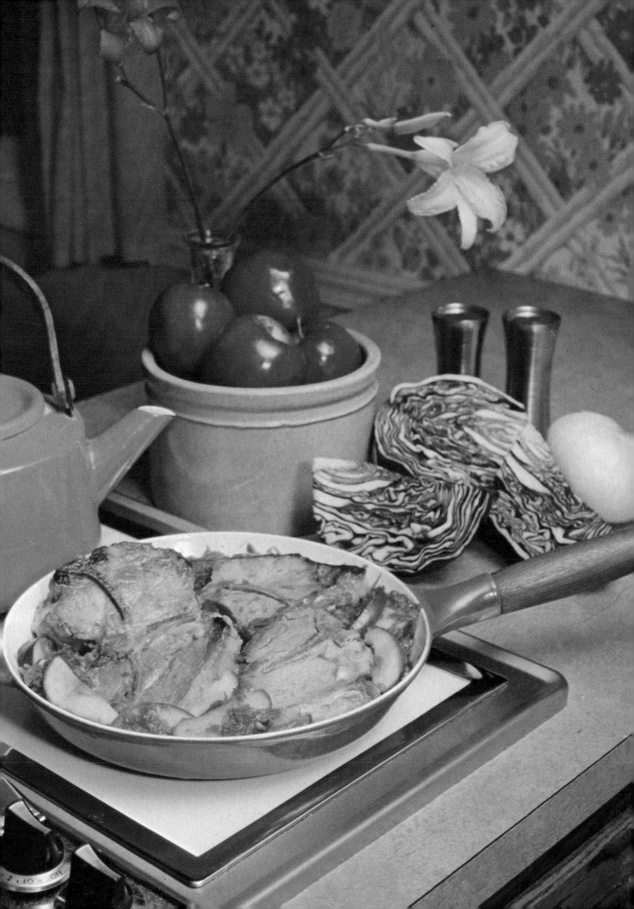

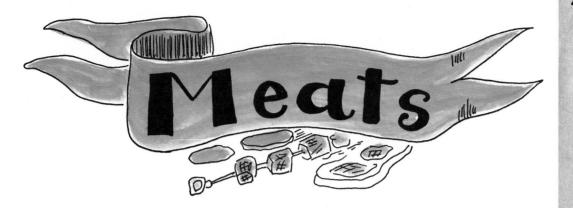

meat

PORK CHOPS
WITH RED CABBAGE

4 loin pork chops, well trimmed
1 large onion, chopped
1 (15-ounce) jar sweet/sour red cabbage
1 small red apple, quartered, cored and sliced

Place pork chops in non-stick pan and brown
  slowly on both sides.
Remove from pan.
Saute onion.
Arrange pork chops over onion.
Cook 30 minutes, turning once.
Lower heat and cover.
Remove chops and keep warm.
Drain liquid from cabbage.
Stir cabbage and apple slices into skillet.
Cook until warmed and apples tender.
Arrange on platter with chops surrounded by
  cabbage.

Serves 4   each: 4 Meat Exchanges
                   1 Vegetable Exchange
                   ½ Fruit Exchange

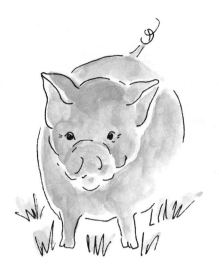

SPANISH PORK CHOPS

6 pork chops, 4 ounces each (all fat trimmed off)
6 teaspoons rice, cooked
6 onion slices
6 tomato slices
salt and pepper to taste

Place chops in baking pan.
Cover each chop with 1 teaspoon rice, 1 slice of onion and 1 slice of tomato.
Season with salt and pepper.
Bake at 350° for 1 hour.

Serves 6   each: 3 Meat Exchanges
                          ½ Bread Exchange

ROUND-UP PORK CHOPS

4-6 lean pork chops
3 green zucchini
2 medium-sized onions, sliced
In a paper sack put:
3 tablespoons flour
1½ teaspoons salt
1½ tablespoons Parmesan cheese
½ teaspoon dillweed
¼ teaspoon pepper

Shake chops in flour mixture in paper sack.
Brown them on both sides in a skillet.
Place onions on the chops.
Add ⅓ cup water, cover and simmer 15 minutes.
Place the sliced, unpeeled zucchini over chops, sprinkle with the left-over flour mixture to which you have added another 3 tablespoons of Parmesan cheese and ½ teaspoon paprika.
Do not stir. Simmer, covered, for another 25 minutes.

Serves 6   each: 3 Meat Exchanges
                          1 Vegetable Exchange
                          ½ Bread Exchange

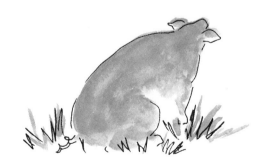

BAKED CHOPS WITH APPLES

4 pork chops, well trimmed
4 small apples, sliced
nutmeg and cinnamon

Put pork chops in flat casserole.
Sprinkle with salt and pepper.
Place sliced apples over chops; sprinkle
   with cinnamon and nutmeg.
Cover with foil and bake at 350° for 1 hour;
   uncover and bake 15 minutes longer.

Serves 4   each: 3 Meat Exchanges
                         1 Fruit Exchange

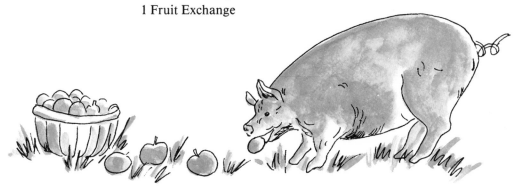

meat

SAUCY PORK CHOPS

4 pork chops
¼ teaspoon salt
¼ teaspoon thyme
1 can chicken rice soup
dash of pepper
2 tablespoons white wine

Brown chops on both sides in skillet.
Season with salt and pepper and thyme.
Add soup and wine; cover and simmer for
   35-45 minutes or bake covered in oven
   at 350° for 50 minutes until tender.
Serves 4   each: 3 Meat Exchanges
                         ½ Bread Exchange

HARVEST PORK CHOPS

6 rib or shoulder pork chops, ½-inch thick
½ cup tomato or V-8 juice
grated rind of ½ orange (optional)
½ cup orange juice
¼ teaspoon salt

Brown chops on both sides in heavy frying
   pan; pour off excess fat.
Combine tomato juice, orange rind, juice and
   salt; pour over and around chops in frying
   pan.
Bake covered at 325° for 1 hour or until
   chops are tender.
Serves 4   each: 4 Meat Exchanges
                         1 Vegetable Exchange
                         ½ Fat Exchange

PORK BELGIAN WITH KRAUT

4 lean center-cut pork chops, each weighing
 5 ounces
salt and pepper
2 cups undrained sauerkraut
1 medium onion, sliced
1 apple, sliced
2 tablespoons chopped parsley
½ teaspoon salt

Spray a large skillet with non-stick vegetable
 cooking spray.

Over medium heat, brown pork chops on
 both sides; sprinkle with salt and pepper.

In an 8-inch square baking dish mix sauerkraut, onions, apple slices, parsley, allspice
 and salt.

Lay pork chops on top of sauerkraut.

Cover and bake at 350° for 1 hour or until
 pork is tender.

Serves 4   each: 4 Meat Exchanges
                    1 Vegetable Exchange
                    ½ Fruit Exchange

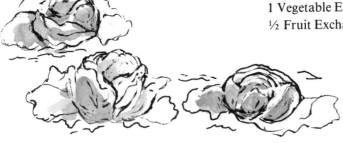

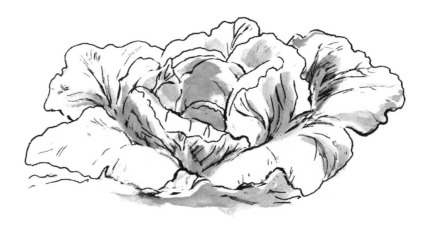

PORK STIR-FRY

1 (10-ounce) package frozen Chinese vege-
tables
3 teaspoons vegetable oil
2 cups thinly sliced cooked pork
¼ cup chopped green onion
soy sauce
1 can chow mein noodles (3 ounces)

Cook vegetables according to package direc-
tions.
Place in a large bowl with 1 tablespoon soy
sauce.
Heat skillet or wok; add oil and meat; stir-fry
until brown.
Add onions, fry 30 seconds.
Stir in vegetables, lifting and turning until
very hot.
Sprinkle with soy sauce and chow mein
noodles.
Serves 4 (without chow mein noodles)
    each: 3 Meat Exchanges
               1 Vegetable Exchange
               1 Fat Exchange
Serves 4 (with chow mein noodles)
    each: 3 Meat Exchanges
               1 Vegetable Exchange
               1 Bread Exchange
               2 Fat Exchanges

meat

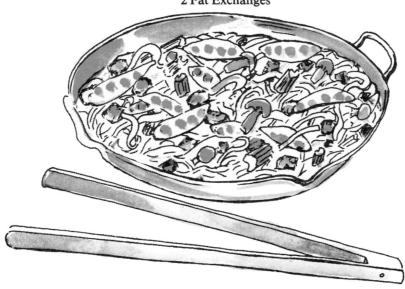

VEAL MARENGO

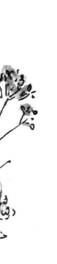

*4 pounds shoulder of veal, boneless, cut into
    1-inch cubes*
salt
flour
1 tablespoon butter
2 tablespoons oil
3 large onions, chopped
1 clove garlic, chopped
1½ cups dry white wine
*1 (10½-ounce) can condensed beef broth, un-
    diluted*
½ cup tomato paste
¼ teaspoon pepper
½ cup chopped parsley
1 pound mushrooms, trimmed and sliced

Sprinkle the veal cubes with salt and roll them
    in the flour.
In a large saucepan or a Dutch oven, heat the
    butter and oil.
Saute onions and garlic for about 5 minutes.
Add veal cubes and continue cooking them
    until lightly browned.
Add wine, beef broth, tomato paste and
    pepper.
Cover and simmer, stirring occasionally until
    the veal is tender (1 hour).
Add the parsley and mushrooms and simmer
    for another 5 minutes.
Thicken the stew with ¼ cup beef broth and
    season to taste with salt.
Serve over rice (optional).
Serves 12   each: 4 Meat Exchanges
                       1 Vegetable Exchange
                       1 Bread Exchange
                       ½ Fat Exchange

try oregano
in meatloaf
for variety ~
or in scrambled eggs ~
    vegetable soups.

ITALIAN VEAL CUTLETS

4 boneless veal cutlets (1 pound)
2 teaspoons shortening
1 (8-ounce) can tomatoes, cut up
1 teaspoon Worcestershire sauce
1 tablespoon snipped parsley
2 teaspoons capers, drained (optional)
¼ teaspoon garlic salt
¼ teaspoon dried oregano leaves, crushed

*rosemary
with basil and lemon juice
on chicken*

Pound veal to ¼-½-inch thickness.
Brown veal quickly in hot shortening.
Blend remaining ingredients and add to meat.
Cover, simmer 35-40 minutes.
Uncover; simmer till tender, about 10 minutes.
To serve, spoon sauce over meat.

Serves 4   each: 3 Meat Exchanges
                     1 Fat Exchange

VEGETABLE-STUFFED VEAL

1½ pounds veal cutlets, cut into 6 thin slices
salt and pepper
¼ teaspoon garlic powder (optional)
⅔ cup finely chopped celery
⅔ cup finely grated carrots
2 tablespoons snipped parsley
½ teaspoon crushed rosemary
1 cup chopped onions
1½ cups beef bouillon
paprika (optional)

Season veal slices with salt, pepper and garlic powder.
Combine celery, carrots, parsley, rosemary and ½ cup chopped onions.
Spoon ⅙ of vegetable mixture onto each veal slice, roll and fasten with toothpicks.
Season to taste with paprika, if desired.
Place meat in roasting pan and add remaining ½ cup onion.
Bake in 425° oven until golden brown (about 30 minutes).
Pour beef bouillon into pan; lower oven temperature to 350° and bake until done, about 45 minutes longer.
Serves 6   each: 4 Meat Exchanges
                    1 Vegetable Exchange

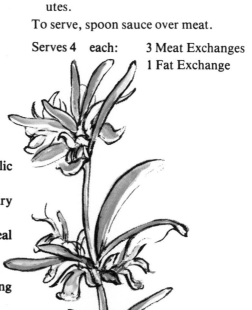

ROSEMARY

meat

LAMB OVEN KABOBS

2 sliced carrots
celery chunks
green pepper squares
mushroom caps
1½ lbs lean boneless lamb cut
    into ¾-inch cubes
1¼ teaspoons salt
⅓ teaspoon pepper
Sauce:
    3 cups tomato juice
    2 tablespoons Worcestershire
        sauce
    ¼ teaspoon whole cloves
    dash of oregano leaves

Parboil the carrots for 10 minutes.
On 4 or 6 individual skewers
    arrange carrot slices, celery
    chunks, green pepper squares,
    mushroom caps and lamb
    cubes.
Place skewers in a single layer in
    a roasting pan.
Sprinkle on all sides with salt and
    pepper.
Combine tomato juice, Worces-
    tershire sauce, cloves and ore-
    gano leaves.
Pour over kabobs.
Bake in 325° oven for 1½ hours
    or until well done.
Baste frequently with pan liquid.
Serves 6
    each: 3 Meat Exchanges
             1 Vegetable Exchange

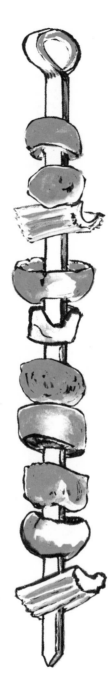

SHISH KABOBS

1½ lb. boneless beef or lamb
2 large tomatoes
2 medium onions
2 medium green peppers
12 bay leaves
12 slices lemon peel
¼ cup diet Italian salad dressing

Cut the meat into 1½-inch cubes,
    trimming off all fat.
Cut each tomato and onion into 6
    wedges, and each green pepper
    into 6 pieces.
On one set of skewers, alternate
    the meat, bay leaves and lemon
    peel.
On a second set of skewers, ar-
    range the tomatoes.
On a third set of skewers alter-
    nate the onion and green
    pepper.
Brush all with the salad dressing.
Grill kabobs (meat, onion and
    green pepper) for 5-7 minutes
    on each side.
Grill tomatoes for 3 minutes on
    each side.
Baste frequently with salad dress-
    ing.
Serves 6
    each: 4 Meat Exchanges
             ½ Vegetable Exchange

QUICK LAMB

1 pound lamb stew
2 large carrots
4 small potatoes
1 (10-ounce) package frozen peas
2 tablespoons olive oil
Salt, pepper, rosemary

Start with peeling and slicing the potatoes
  (and carrots).
Place on the bottom of roasting pan; add peas.
Pour on oil; add salt and pepper.
Place meat on top of vegetables. Add rose-
  mary to taste. Do not cover.
Bake at 375° about 1½ hours.

Serves 4   each: 4 Meat Exchanges
                   1 Bread Exchange
                   2 Vegetable Exchanges
                   2 Fat Exchanges

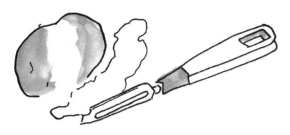

OVEN BEEF STEW

2 pounds round steak
1 medium onion, chopped
3 stalks celery, sliced
2 teaspoons salt
2 tablespoons tapioca
6 carrots, sliced
½ cup tomato juice

Place vegetables over meat in 9x13-inch
  baking dish.
Sprinkle salt and tapioca over vegetables and
  meat.
Pour tomato juice over top.
Cover with foil and bake at 250° for 4 hours.
Serves 6   each: 4 Meat Exchanges
                   2 Vegetable Exchanges
                   2 Fat Exchanges

meat

MEAL-IN-ONE CASSEROLE

1 pound lean ground beef
1 large carrot, sliced
1 large onion, sliced
½ box frozen peas
½ can vegetable soup
⅓ cup cracker crumbs
⅓ cup tapioca
salt and pepper to taste

Combine all ingredients, stirring to mix well.
Put into 2-quart baking dish.
Bake for 2 hours at 375°.

Serves 6   each: 2 Meat Exchanges
                   1 Bread Exchange
                   1 Vegetable Exchange

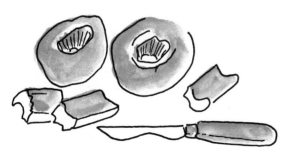

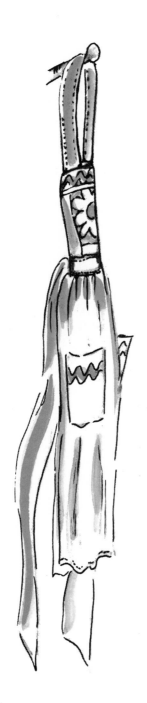

STIR-FRIED BEEF WITH BROCCOLI

1 pound flank steak
2 tablespoons soy sauce
1 garlic clove, minced
1 tablespoon cornstarch
¼ cup water
1 beef bouillon cube, mashed
1 tablespoon salt
1 bunch broccoli, cut into flowerettes
1 cup thinly sliced celery
1 tablespoon salad oil
1 tablespoon pimento, cut into strips

Cut flank steak into thirds lengthwise.
Freeze about 30 minutes for easier slicing.
Slice steak across the grain into very thin diagonal pieces.
In medium bowl combine soy sauce and garlic.
Add beef and toss until well coated.
Marinate for 30 minutes.
In small cup combine cornstarch, water and bouillon.
In large saucepan bring 3 quarts water and 1 tablespoon salt to boil.
Blanch broccoli flowerettes for one minute.
Add celery, continue to blanch both for one more minute; drain.
In a medium skillet, heat oil until hot but not smoking.
Add beef and cook, stirring quickly and frequently, until beef loses its pink color, about three minutes.
Stir in cornstarch mixture and cook one minute.
Add blanched vegetables and pimento and cook for one more minute or until mixture is hot.

Serves 4   each: 4 Meat Exchanges
                          2 Vegetable Exchanges
                          ½ Fat Exchange

OVEN STEAK DINNER

1½ pounds round steak
1 envelope onion soup mix
4 small carrots, quartered
2 stalks celery, cut in sticks
3-4 medium potatoes, halved
1 tablespoon butter
½ teaspoon salt

Place meat in center of 3-foot length of foil.
Sprinkle meat with dry soup mix; cover with
   vegetables; dot with butter and sprinkle
   with salt.
Fold foil and seal securely to hold in juices.
Place on baking sheet, and bake at 350° for
   1½ hours or until done.

Serves 6   each: 3 Meat Exchanges
                      1 Bread Exchange
                      2 Vegetable Exchanges
                      2 Fat Exchanges

STUFFED FLANK STEAK

1 pound flank steak, scored
4 slices white bread, made into crumbs
1 (4-5 ounce) can mushrooms, finely chopped
½ green pepper, finely minced
2 stalks celery, finely minced
1 teaspoon poultry seasoning
1 teaspoon sage
½ teaspoon garlic powder
¼-½ cup chicken bouillon to moisten
salt and pepper to taste

Roll steak in small amount of flour and
   brown in non-stick pan.
Spread stuffing over steak and roll as for
   a jelly roll.
Place in oven with ½ cup water and bake
   at 350° for 1½ hours or till tender.

Serves 4   each: 4 Meat Exchanges
                      1 Bread Exchange
                      1 Vegetable Exchange

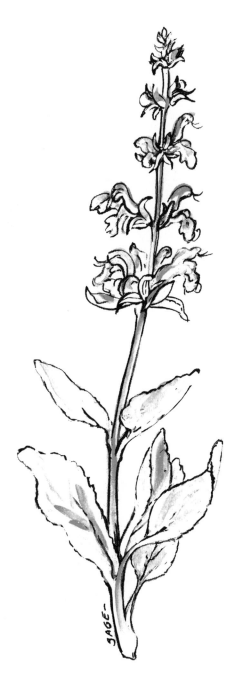

SAGE

sage is good
in stuffings~
or try a pinch
in cornbread

meat

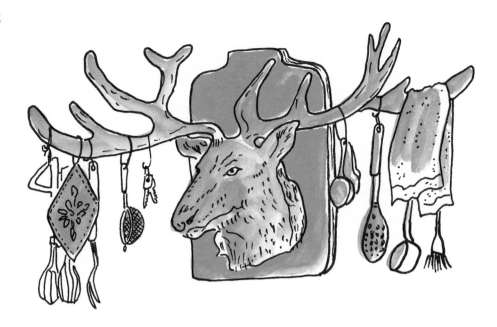

VENISON ROAST

Cover the roast with buttermilk.

Marinate in refrigerator overnight.

Drain and wipe dry.

Salt and pepper, and then rub with mashed garlic.

Put slices of onion over the top of the roast and cover with bacon or thinly-sliced salt pork.

Roast in preheated 350° oven for 30 minutes for each pound or until meat thermometer registers the degree of doneness you like.

Since venison is a dry meat, take these precautions if you want gravy:

for a 4-pound roast, mix 2 cups water, ¼ cup cider vinegar, 1 cup tomato juice, 2 tablespoons sugar and 2 cups sliced celery, and put into the pan with the roasting venison.

When the meat is done, put on platter and keep warm.

Skim fat from pan juices and serve.

Add salt and pepper.

Serves 15   each: 4 Meat Exchanges
     Gravy, ½ cup: 1 Vegetable Exchange

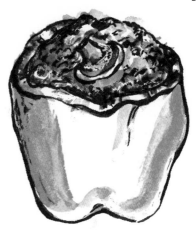

BEEF-CABBAGE CASSEROLE

1 pound lean ground beef
1 small minced onion
4 ounces tomato sauce
4-7 ounces tomato juice
⅛ teaspoon cinnamon
⅛ teaspoon ground cloves
4 cups shredded cabbage

Brown meat and drain all fat; blot meat well
in paper toweling.
Mix onion, tomato sauce and juice, cinna-
mon and cloves, and add to beef.
Using half of total amount, make a bed of
cabbage in a 2-quart casserole.
Top cabbage with meat mixture and repeat
layers of cabbage and meat mixture.
Cover and bake at 350° for 45 minutes.
Serves 4   each: 4 Meat Exchanges
                     2 Vegetable Exchanges
                     ½ Fat Exchange

STUFFED PEPPER

1 green pepper, blanched
4 ounces lean ground beef
¼ cup tomato sauce
¼ cup diced mushrooms
1 teaspoon onion flakes
salt and pepper to taste
dash of oregano
dash of basil

Brown the beef, mix with other ingredients
and fill the pepper.
Place in individual baking dish in one inch of
water.
Bake for 15 minutes at 350°.
Serves 1   each: 4 Meat Exchanges
                     1 Bread Exchanges
                     2 Vegetable Exchanges

meat

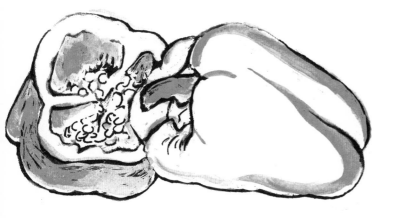

130

HUNGARIAN SKILLET RAGOUT

1 pound top round steak, lean and boneless,
  cut in 2-inch cubes
1 cup tomato juice
1 large onion
1 clove garlic, minced
1 teaspoon paprika
1 teaspoon caraway seeds
pinch of red cayenne pepper
salt and pepper to taste
2 ribs celery, sliced
2 carrots, scraped and sliced
2 potatoes, peeled and sliced
1 teaspoon cornstarch
¼ cup cold water

In a non-stick pan, brown meat slowly over
  moderate heat.
Drain all fat.
Add tomato juice, onion, garlic, paprika,
  caraway, cayenne, salt and pepper.
Cover and simmer until meat is tender, about
  45-60 minutes.
Stir in vegetables. Cover and simmer until
  potatoes are tender — about 20 minutes.
Combine cornstarch with water and stir into
  simmering skillet until thickened.

Serves 4   each: 3 Meat Exchanges
   2 Vegetable Exchanges
   1 Bread Exchange

TAMALE PIE

1 pound ground beef
2 onions, diced
1 clove garlic, mashed
1 teaspoon salt
½ teaspoon chili powder
1 large can of tomatoes
½ package cornbread mix

Brown together beef, onions, garlic, salt and
  chili powder.
Add tomatoes.
Place in 1½-quart casserole.
Mix one-half recipe of cornbread batter ac-
  cording to directions on package.
Spread cornbread over the top of the meat
  mixture.
Bake at 400° for 35 minutes.

Serves 4   each: 4 Meat Exchanges
   2 Bread Exchanges
   1 Vegetable Exchange
   2 Fat Exchanges

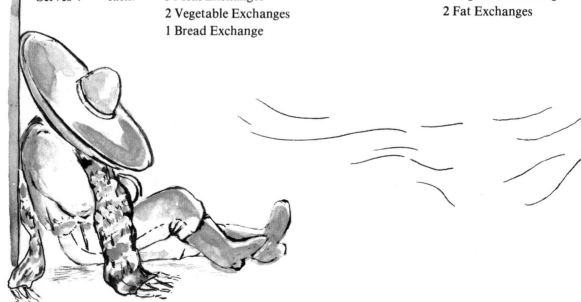

POT ROAST SUPREME

3 pounds chuck roast of beef
1 large onion, sliced
lemon pepper
1 package brown gravy mix
3 tablespoons red wine
10 medium potatoes
*10 medium carrots, pared and cut in thick
   slices*

Arrange beef in a large casserole.
Place onion on beef.
Sprinkle with lemon pepper and gravy mix.
Pour wine over top.
Cover and roast in 350° oven.
Add carrots and potatoes the last 45-60 min-
   utes of cooking.
Total time: 2½-3 hours.

4 ounces meat	=	4 Meat Exchanges
1 medium potato	=	1 Bread Exchange
½ cup carrots	=	1 Vegetable Exchange

No gravy.

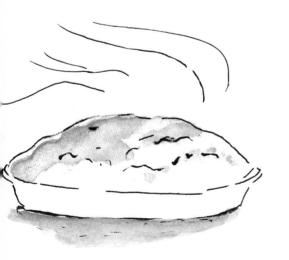

SESAME LIVER SAUTE

2 large onions, thinly sliced
1 pound baby beef liver
3 tablespoons lemon juice
½ cup sesame seed

Saute onions in small amount of butter or
   margarine until limp and golden.
Cut liver in ½-1 inch strips.
Pour lemon juice over liver pieces and let
   stand for 10 minutes.
When onions are cooked, remove from pan
   and keep warm.
Drain liver strips; dredge each in sesame seed
   and saute until liver is browned on all sides
   (3-5 minutes).
Turn into serving dish and top with onions.

Serves 4   each: 4 Meat Exchanges
                     1 Vegetable Exchange
                     1 Bread Exchange

BREADED LIVER

1 pound baby beef liver
⅓ cup skim milk powder
1 teaspoon salt
1 teaspoon onion salt
1 teaspoon oregano leaves
2 tablespoons chicken broth

Combine milk powder and seasonings.
Dip liver into milk mixture.
Heat broth in non-stick pan; add liver and
   cook for 5 minutes or until browned on
   both sides and cooked throughout.

Serves 4   each: 4 Meat Exchanges
                     ¼ Milk Exchange

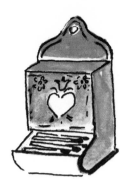

DIET LASAGNA

1 pound ground round
¼ cup chopped onion
1 (8-ounce) can tomato puree
½ teaspoon basil
1 teaspoon parsley
1 teaspoon oregano
1 teaspoon garlic salt
dash pepper
1 (4-ounce) can mushrooms, drained
4 ounces mozzarella cheese, cut in strips
1 (10-ounce) package frozen chopped spinach
6 ounces cottage cheese

Saute beef and onions.
Drain off fat.
Add puree, basil, parsley, oregano, salt, pepper and mushrooms.
Thaw spinach and squeeze out water.
Combine spinach and cottage cheese.
In 9-inch square or 7x11-inch dish, arrange in layers: spinach mixture, meat mixture and cheese.
Repeat, ending with cheese.
Bake at 375° for 15-20 minutes or until hot and bubbly.
Serves 6   each: 3 Meat Exchanges
                        1 Vegetable Exchanges
                        2 Fat Exchanges

STUFFED SHELLS

8 jumbo macaroni shells
1½ cups tomato puree
1 teaspoon basil, crushed
1 teaspoon salt
½ pound lean ground beef
1 small onion, chopped
1 garlic clove, minced
1 package frozen, chopped spinach, thawed and drained
2 tablespoons grated Parmesan cheese
½ cup low fat cottage cheese

Cook shells for 20 minutes; drain.
In small bowl combine tomato puree, basil and salt; set aside.
In non-stick skillet, brown ground beef with onion and garlic; drain.
Preheat oven to 350°.
To meat in skillet, add ⅓ cup tomato mixture, spinach, cheeses and ¼ teaspoon salt.
Fill each cooked shell with ¼ cup of the meat mixture.
Place shells in 9-inch square pan.
Combine remaining meat mixture with sauce and pour over shells.
Cover with foil and bake 40-45 minutes until hot and bubbly.
Serves 6   each: 2 Meat Exchanges
                        2 Bread Exchanges
                        1 Vegetable Exchange
                        1 Fat Exchange

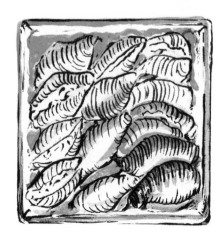

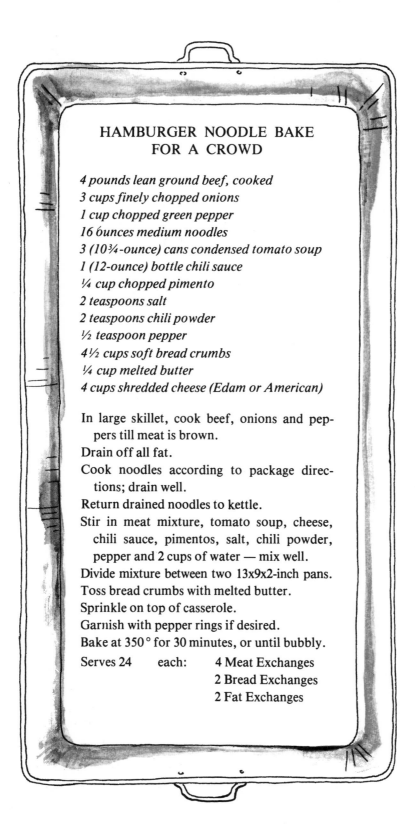

HAMBURGER NOODLE BAKE
FOR A CROWD

4 pounds lean ground beef, cooked
3 cups finely chopped onions
1 cup chopped green pepper
16 6unces medium noodles
3 (10¾-ounce) cans condensed tomato soup
1 (12-ounce) bottle chili sauce
¼ cup chopped pimento
2 teaspoons salt
2 teaspoons chili powder
½ teaspoon pepper
4½ cups soft bread crumbs
¼ cup melted butter
4 cups shredded cheese (Edam or American)

In large skillet, cook beef, onions and peppers till meat is brown.

Drain off all fat.

Cook noodles according to package directions; drain well.

Return drained noodles to kettle.

Stir in meat mixture, tomato soup, cheese, chili sauce, pimentos, salt, chili powder, pepper and 2 cups of water — mix well.

Divide mixture between two 13x9x2-inch pans.

Toss bread crumbs with melted butter.

Sprinkle on top of casserole.

Garnish with pepper rings if desired.

Bake at 350° for 30 minutes, or until bubbly.

Serves 24   each: 4 Meat Exchanges
2 Bread Exchanges
2 Fat Exchanges

meat

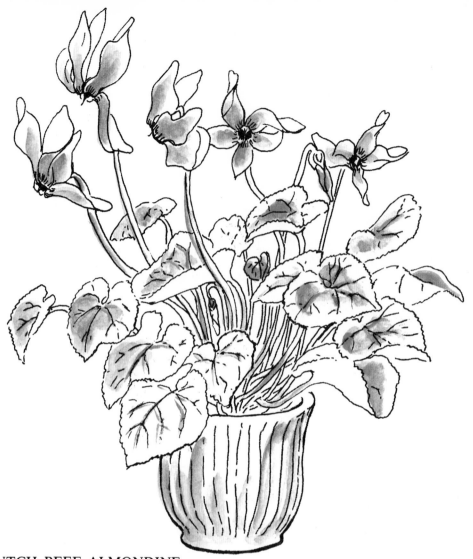

DUTCH BEEF ALMONDINE

⅓ cup flour

¼ teaspoon each: cloves, ginger, curry powder, garlic salt, pepper

1½ pounds 1-inch thick round steak

½ teaspoon salt

¼ cup salad oil

2 cups boiling water

2 tablespoons butter

¼ cup slivered almonds

1 (4-ounce) can mushrooms

1 cup sour pie cherries, drained

Combine flour with all seasonings. Cut meat into 1-inch cubes; dredge in seasoned flour.

Cut meat into 1-inch cubes; dredge in seasoned flour.

Brown meat in hot oil.

Pour water on browned meat and simmer 2 hours.

Saute almonds; add mushrooms, almonds and cherries to meat and heat 10 minutes.

(Add water if gravy is too thick.)

Spoon over rice or noodles (optional).

Garnish with sour cream (optional).

(Can be made ahead and frozen or refrigerated.)

Serves 6   each: 4 Meat Exchanges
                       2 Fat Exchanges
                       ½ Bread Exchange

ZUCCHINI BEEF BOATS

4 medium zucchini
1 pound ground round
1 medium onion, chopped
½ cup chopped celery
1 (8- ounce) can tomato sauce
½ cup chopped mushrooms
¾ teaspoon salt
½ teaspoon oregano
¼ teaspoon pepper
8 ounces mozzarella cheese
1 clove garlic, minced

Cut zucchini in half lengthwise; remove seeds and pulp and steam boats for 5-10 minutes.

drain off excess fat.

Brown ground round in a non-stick pan.

Combine remaining ingredients, except mozzarella, and blend with meat.

Fill zucchini boats and bake 30 minutes at 350°.

Top with Mozzarella for the last 5 minutes.

Serves 8   each: 2 Meat Exchanges
2 Vegetable Exchanges
1 Fat Exchange

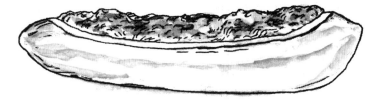

136

POLYNESIAN SANDWICH

1 ounce sliced ham
1 slice bread
1 ounce cheese (American, Swiss or your favorite)
1 pineapple ring

Butter bread on one side with ½ teaspoon butter and place on broiler.

Add ham and pineapple ring to each sandwich and place under broiler to heat through.

Place cheese on sandwich and broil until melted.

Serves 1	2 Meat Exchanges
	1 Bread Exchange
	1 fat Exchange
	1 Fruit Exchange

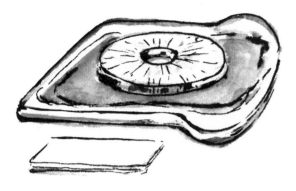

APPLESAUCE MEATLOAF

2 pounds ground round
1 cup unsweetened applesauce
1 onion, finely diced
1 green pepper, finely diced
6 slices whole grain bread, crumbled
1 egg
2 teaspoons salt
pepper to taste
½ cup tomato sauce

Preheat oven to 350°.
Combine all ingredients except tomato sauce.
Knead mixture with hands until well blended.
Pack into loaf pan.
Pour tomato sauce over top of loaf.
Bake for 2 hours.
Turn out of pan, slice and serve.
For Crock-Pot: Pack into bottom of pot.
Pour tomato sauce over the top.
Cover and cook on high for 1 hour.
Then turn to low and cook for 6-8 hours.
Lift out of pot; slice and serve.

Serves 8	each:	4 Meat Exchanges
		1 Bread Exchange
		½ Fruit Exchange

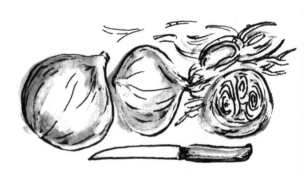

HAMBURGER STUFFED ROLLS

2 ounces lean ground beef
garlic powder
salt and pepper
crescent roll

Brown meat and season to taste.
Drain off fat.
Roll into a crescent roll.
Bake 350° for 10-20 minutes.

Serves 1	2 Meat Exchanges
	1 Bread Exchange
	1 Fat Exchange

REUBEN SANDWICH

1 ounce canned corned beef
1 finely chopped dill pickle
¼ cup drained sauerkraut
1 ounce Swiss cheese
1 slice onion

Spread slice of rye bread with corned beef.
Mix pickle with sauerkraut.
Place on bread.
Top with onion and cheese.
Heat under broiler until cheese melts.
Serves 1   2 Meat Exchanges
                1 Vegetable Exchange
                1 Bread Exchange
                1 Fat Exchange

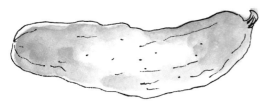

GRILLED BEEF SANDWICHES

2 tablespoons prepared horseradish
dash pepper
⅓ cup margarine or butter
12 slices white bread
12 thin slices cooked, leftover roast beef
6 slices Swiss cheese

Stir horseradish and pepper into margarine or
    butter.
Spread on both sides of each slice of bread.
Top half of slices with roast beef and cheese,
    put remaining slice of bread on top.
Over medium low heat brown the sandwiches
    on both sides in a skillet till cheese melts.
Serves 6   each: 2 Meat Exchanges
                    2 Bread Exchanges
                    3 Fat Exchanges

HAM STUFFED ROLLS

2 cups finely chopped boiled ham
2 hard cooked eggs, finely chopped
2 tablespoons minced green onions
2 tablespoons minced green pepper
1 teaspoon prepared mustard
1 tablespoon pickle relish
¼ cup low-calorie mayonnaise
6 medium-size French rolls
½ cup shredded Swiss cheese

Combine first seven ingredients.
Cut off top of rolls; scoop out and fill with
    ham mixture.
Place in 7½ x 12-inch baking dish.
Sprinkle with cheese.
Heat at 350° for 20 minutes.
Serves 6   each: 2 Meat Exchanges
                         1 Bread Exchange
                         1 Vegetable Exchange
                         3 Fat Exchanges

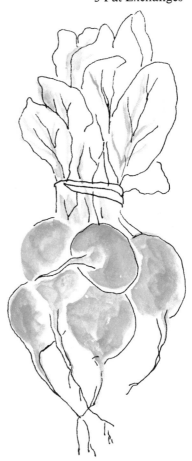

meat

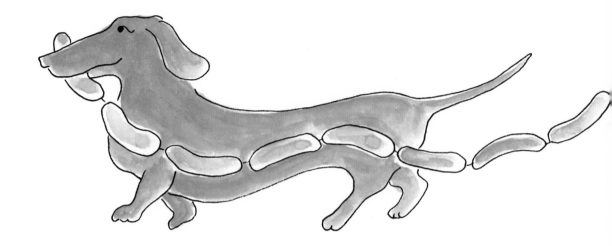

OPEN-FACED HOT DOG
REUBENS

4 slices rye bread, toasted
4 chicken hot dogs, boiled and split
1 can sauerkraut, drained
4 tablespoons low-calorie Russian dressing
4 (1-ounce) slices Swiss cheese

Layer sandwich in the above order.
Put under broiler.
Serving suggestion: cut in small pieces and
  serve as hors d'oeuvres.
4 sandwiches
        each: 2 Meat Exchanges
                  1 Bread Exchange
                  1 Vegetable Exchange
                  2 Fat Exchanges

CHEESE-FRANK SANDWICH

6 (1 ounce each) cheese slices
6 frankfurters, thinly sliced
6 slices bread

Arrange cheese on bread and top with sliced
   frankfurters.
Place under broiler and broil lightly.

Serves 6	each:	2 Meat Exchanges
		1 Bread Exchange
		2 Fat Exchanges

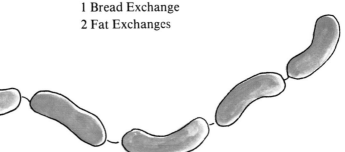

STUFFED BAKED FRANKS

1 pound chicken frankfurters
¼ cup finely chopped onions
1 tablespoon butter or margarine
2 cups herb-seasoned stuffing mix
¼ cup catsup
1 tablespoon sweet pickle relish
3 slices mozzarella cheese

Cut franks lengthwise almost to opposite side.
Cook onions in butter till tender but not
   brown.
Combine stuffing mix, onion, catsup, pickle
   relish and ¾ cup water; mix well.
Mound stuffing atop franks.
Place on baking sheet.
Bake at 400° until heated, 10-12 minutes.
Cut cheese slices in strips, place atop franks;
   return to oven and cook until cheese melts,
   about 3 minutes.

Serves 6	each:	2 Meat Exchanges
		½ Bread Exchange
		2 Fat Exchanges

meat

My son, eat honey, for it is good, and the drippings of the honeycomb are sweet to your taste.

Proverbs 24:13

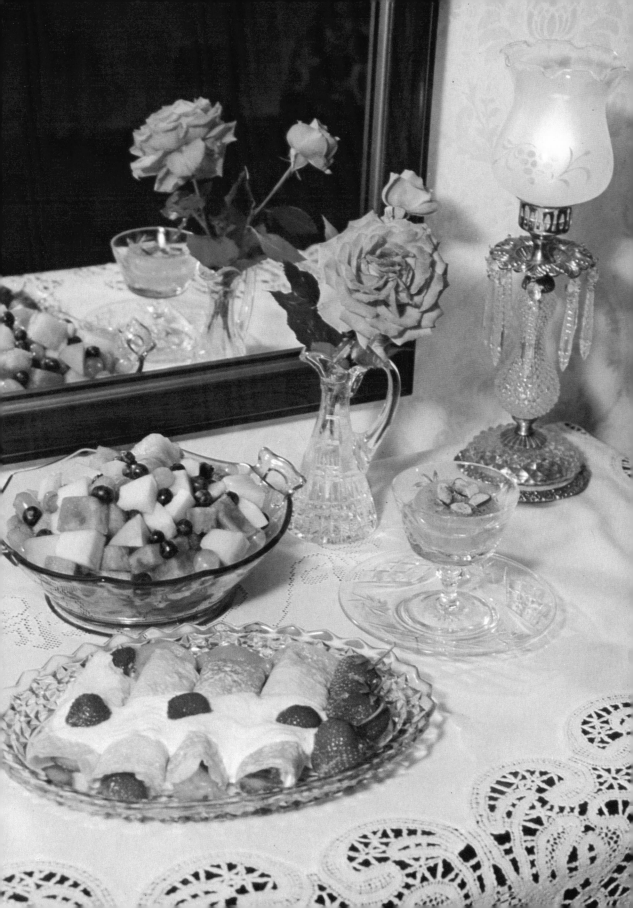

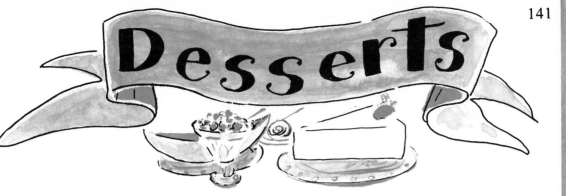

STRAWBERRY CREPES

1 pint fresh strawberries, sliced
2 ripe soft peaches, peeled and sliced
¼ cup orange juice
1 cup plain low-fat yogurt
½ cup sour cream or low-fat sour cream dressing
1 teaspoon vanilla
12 crepes

Combine the strawberries, peaches and orange juice, and chill several hours to blend the flavors.

In a separate bowl blend the yogurt, sour cream and vanilla and chill.

Fill crepes with fruit mix and a little of the yogurt-cream mix.

Roll up and top with additional yogurt-cream.

Serves 6   each serving of 2 crepes equals
    1 Bread Exchange
    1 Fruit Exchange
    ½ Milk Exchange

For crepe recipe, see page 87.

APPLE COMPOTE

4 small apples, unpeeled and sliced
2 tablespoons raisins
⅓ cup unsweetened pineapple juice
½ teaspoon cinnamon
⅛ teaspoon nutmeg

Place all ingredients in saucepan and bring to
  a boil.
Simmer until apples are tender but still firm.
Serves 6   each: 1 Fruit Exchange

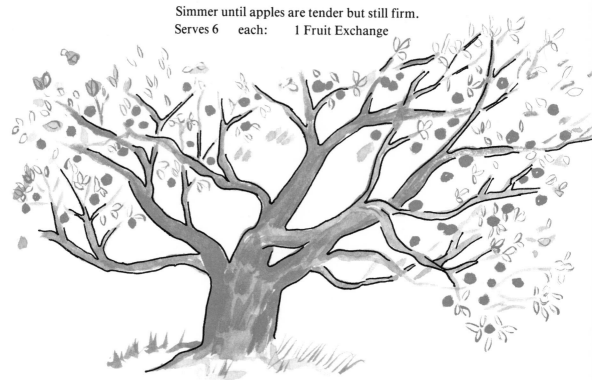

BAKED APPLE

2-inch apples: Pippin, Winesap, Jonathan,
McIntosh or Cortland

Core, but don't cut all the way through apple
  (so it will hold liquid).
Peel the top ⅓ of the apple.
Place apple in a baking dish.
In apple hole, sprinkle cinnamon and ¼ cup
  apple juice.
Bake 20 minutes at 350°.
Serves 1   1½ Fruit Exchanges

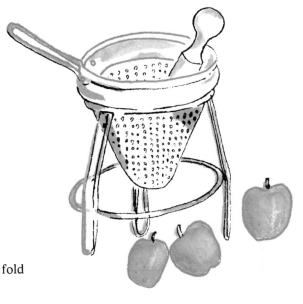

APPLESAUCE DESSERT

6 ounces unsweetened applesauce
1 package diet gelatin
1 cup low-calorie ginger ale

Bring ½ cup ginger ale to boiling.
Dissolve gelatin in hot ginger ale.
Mix remaining ingredients together and fold
   into gelatin mixture.
Refrigerate until set.
Serves 2   each: 1 Fruit Exchange

APPLESAUCE
(Unsweetened)

3 medium-size apples (approximately one
   pound)
⅓-⅔ cup unsweetened apple juice
   (depending on juiciness of apples)
½ teaspoon cinnamon
⅛ teaspoon nutmeg (optional)

Wash and peel apples and remove core.
Place in saucepan.
Add juice to the apples.
Cover pan tightly and simmer for 5-10 min-
   utes or until apples are tender.
Add cinnamon. Sauce will be chunky in con-
   sistency.
Serves 5   each: 1½ Fruit Exchanges

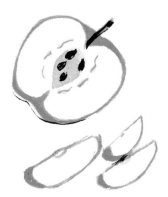

dessert

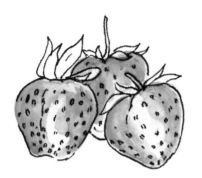

FRESH FRUIT COMPOTE

1 cup white grape juice
1 teaspoon grated orange rind
1 pint whole strawberries, hulled
2 cups seedless green grapes
2 cups honeydew melon balls
2 cups cantaloupe balls
1 cup blueberries

Combine fruits with grape juice.
Chill 1-2 hours.
Serves 12   each: 1 Fruit Exchange

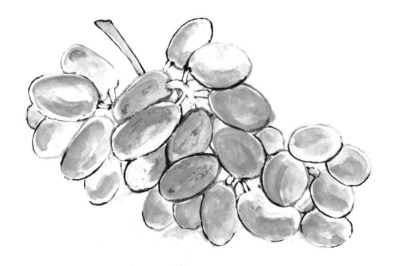

a very
pretty
dessert
or
appetizer ~
slice of honeydew melon
garnished with lime slices.
Drizzle the lime juice on melon.

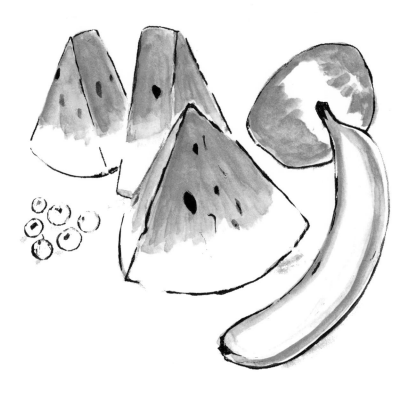

FRUIT SALAD

1 banana
1 apple
1 pear
1 orange
1 cup strawberries
3 tablespoons honey
1 teaspoon lemon juice

Wash and cut fruit.
Combine all cut up fruit, honey and lemon
  juice.
Chill and serve.
Serves 8   each: 1 Fruit Exchange

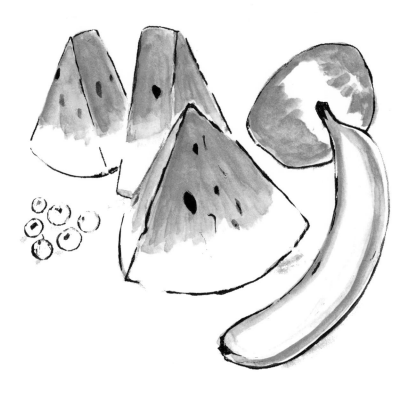

dessert

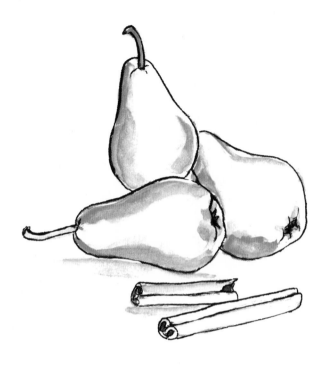

PEACH PIE

6 peach halves
1 cup diet whipped topping
2 envelopes diet cherry gelatin

Place peach halves round-side-up in 9-inch pie plate.
Cover with whipped topping.
Prepare gelatin according to directions and chill until consistency of egg whites.
Spread gently over topping and peaches to cover completely.
Chill until firm.
Cut as a pie.

Serves 6   each: ½ Fruit Exchange
                   ½ Fat Exchange

BAKED CRIMSON PEARS

4 fresh medium pears
1 cup low-calorie cranberry juice cocktail
3 inch cinnamon sticks
10 drops red food coloring

Peel, halve and core pears; place in 1-quart casserole.
Mix cranberry juice, cinnamon and food coloring; bring to boiling.
Pour over pears; bake uncovered for 10 minutes at 350°.
Turn pears; bake uncovered until tender, 7-10 minutes more.
Remove cinnamon sticks.
Serve with juice.

Serves 8   each: 2 Fruit Exchanges

BAKED PEACH HALF

4 dietetic-packed peach-halves
2 teaspoons butter
slivered almonds
nutmeg

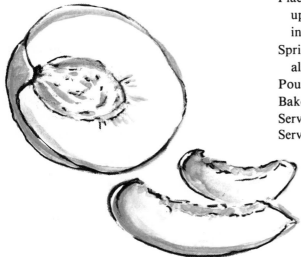

Heat oven to 425°.
Place four drained peach-halves hollow-side-
up in a baking dish with ½ teaspoon butter
in each.
Sprinkle with nutmeg and toasted slivered
almonds.
Pour a little fruit juice around the peaches.
Bake 12 minutes.
Serve warm or cold.
Serves 4   each: 1 Fruit Exchange
                      1 Fat Exchange

PEACH PARFAIT

1 envelope diet raspberry-flavored gelatin
few drops almond extract
1½ cups water
1 pound can dietetic-pack peaches, drained
  and chopped
⅓ cup chilled evaporated skim milk

Prepare gelatin according to directions on
  package, but use only 1½ cups water.
Mix peaches with 1 cup gelatin until partially
  set.
Chill remaining gelatin until partially set.
Add evaporated milk and almond extract
  to the gelatin without fruit.
Whip till fluffy.
Alternate the 2 gelatin mixtures in parfait
  glasses ending with whipped gelatin.
Serves 6   each: 1 Fruit Exchange

dessert

GINGER FRUIT COCKTAIL

½ cup pineapple cubes
½ cup orange sections
½ cups peach cubes
½ cup fresh strawberries, sliced
1 cup low-calorie ginger ale

Combine and serve chilled in attractive dish;
    garnish with mint.

Serves 4   each: 1 Fruit Exchange

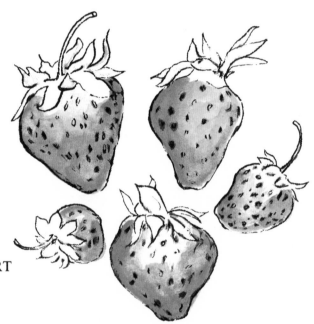

TWO-TONE MOLDED DESSERT

1 envelope diet strawberry gelatin
1 envelope diet lime gelatin
2 envelopes diet whipped topping mix
1 cup strawberries
1 cup drained unsweetened pineapple

Make strawberry gelatin according to pack-
    age directions.
Add berries and chill.
Make lime gelatin according to package direc-
    tions; add pineapple and chill.
Make 2 packages diet whipped topping
    according to directions; fold ½ into each
bowl of gelatin with fruit when almost firm.
Layer lime and strawberry gelatins in mold.
Chill until firm.
Serves 8   each: 1 Fruit Exchange

STRAWBERRY SPONGE

1 envelope unflavored gelatin
½ cup cold water
1 tablespoon artificial sweetener
1½ teaspoons lemon juice
1 pint strawberries
2 egg whites

Soften gelatin in water in top of double
  boiler.
Add sweetener and lemon juice.
Heat, stirring until gelatin dissolves.
Remove from heat and add crushed berries.
Let stand until thick, then beat until light and
  fluffy.
Beat egg whites until stiff and fold in gelatin.
Spoon into 6 individual molds.
Chill.
Serves 6   each: ½ Fruit Exchange

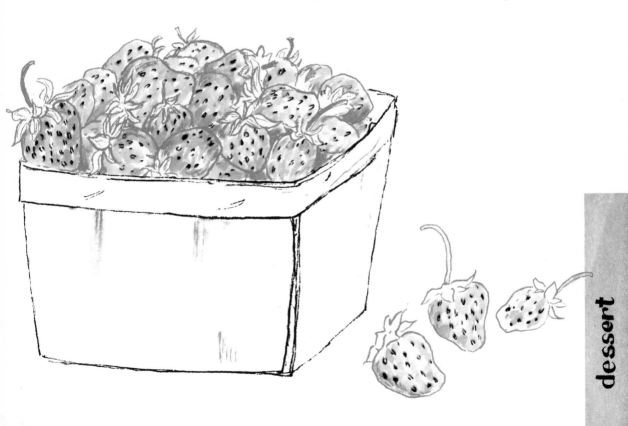

dessert

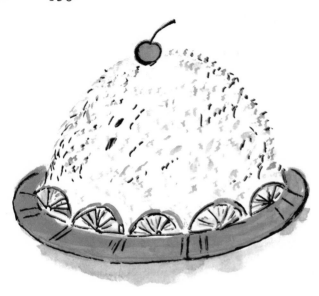

SNOWBALL CAKE

2 tablespoons unflavored gelatin
1 cup orange juice
1 teaspoon lemon juice
½ cup granulated sugar
dash salt
4 cups diet whipped topping
1 large angel food cake ring
¼ cup flaked coconut

Line a medium bowl with waxed paper.
In separate bowl, mix together gelatin and 4 tablespoons of water until dissolved.
Add 1 cup boiling water, orange juice, lemon juice, sugar and salt.
Mix and chill until syrupy.
Add 3 cups of whipped topping to chilled gelatin.
Break angel food cake into bite-sized cubes.
Fold Cake into gelatin mixture.
Pour into wax paper-lined bowl.
Chill until firm.
Turn out onto plate and frost with remaining whipped topping, coconut and a cherry.
Serves 15   each: 2 Bread Exchanges
1 Fruit Exchange
1 Fat Exchange

HAWAIIAN ICE

1 (6-ounce) can frozen orange-pineapple juice
¾ cup unsweetened apple juice
¾ cup cold water
1½ teaspoons sugar substitute (optional)
¼ cup skim milk powder

Combine liquids and sweetener, stirring until dissolved.
Add dry milk and blend well.
Pour into chilled refrigerator tray.
Place in freezer for 45-60 minutes until ice begins to freeze.
Turn ice into chilled mixer bowl and beat until fluffy but not melted.
Return to freezer and continue to freeze until almost set.
Repeat beating procedure.
Keep in freezer compartment until needed.
Serves 4   each: 1 Fruit Exchange

LEMON-ORANGE GELATIN

1 envelope unflavored gelatin
½ cup cold water
½ cup boiling water
2 tablespoons honey
pinch of salt
grated rind of 1 lemon
½ cup lemon juice
½ cup orange juice
3 medium-size oranges, peeled and separated into segments

Soften gelatin in cold water; combine with boiling water, stirring until gelatin is dissolved.
Add honey, salt, lemon rind and juices.
Chill in refrigerator until partially set.
Fold in oranges and continue to chill until completely set.
Serves 10   each: 1 Fruit Exchange

FROZEN PINEAPPLE DESSERT

1 envelope unflavored gelatin
2 cups skim milk
1½ teaspoons coconut extract
1½ teaspoons butter extract
1 (15¼-ounce) can crushed pineapple packed
  in its own juice (reserve juice)

Dissolve gelatin in ½ cup water plus 1 table-
  spoon pineapple juice and heat until gelatin
  dissolves.
Cool slightly.
Add remaining ingredients and mix well.
Spread in 8x8 foil-lined pan and freeze.
Cut into squares and garnish with mint leaves
  or lime slices.
Serves 6   each: 1 Fruit Exchange
                      1 Milk Exchange

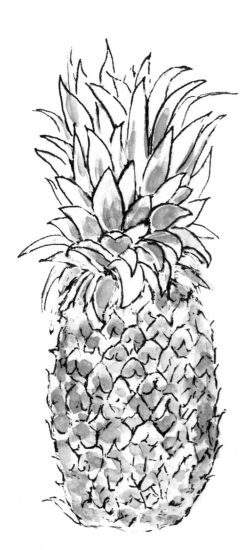

PINEAPPLE DELIGHT

1 fresh pineapple
½ cup fresh pitted cherries
1 cup cantaloupe, cut in small squares

With a sharp knife remove top of pineapple.
Remove insides by running sharp knife
  around the edges.
Cut in small wedges.
Combine with cherries and melon squares.
Scoop fruit into hollowed pineapple shell.
Serves 10   each: 1 Fruit Exchange

dessert

LIME-PINEAPPLE FOAM

1 package diet lime-flavored gelatin
½ cup canned pineapple juice
2 cups crushed ice

Heat pineapple juice to boiling point and
   pour into blender with the lime gelatin.
Cover and blend at high speed for 20 seconds.
Add crushed ice.
Cover and blend for 30 seconds more.
Pour into 2-cup mold and chill until firm.
Serves 2   each: ½ Fruit Exchange

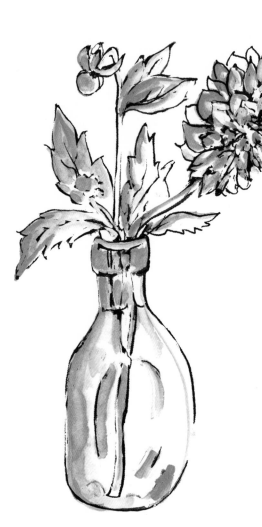

FROZEN FRUIT DESSERT

1 package unflavored gelatin
artificial sweetener to taste
½ cup boiling water
⅔ cup skim milk powder
1 cup frozen fruit

Put enough cold water in blender to cover
   blades.
Sprinkle gelatin over water.
Let soften for a few minutes.
Add sweetener and flavoring if desired.
Add boiling water and blend.
Then blend in milk.
As blender runs at high speed, gradually add
   cut frozen fruit.
(If mixture becomes too thick, add more boil-
   ing water.)
Place in individual serving dishes.

Serves 2   each: 1 Fruit Exchange
                      1 Milk Exchange

RICE MERINGUE PUDDING

⅓ cup long grain rice
2 beaten egg yolks
1 egg white
1 cup skim milk
2 tablespoons sugar
2 tablespoons water
⅛ teaspoon cinnamon
½ teaspoon vanilla
1 egg white
1 tablespoon sugar

Cook rice according to package directions and set aside.

In small saucepan combine egg yolks, 1 egg white, milk, 2 tablespoons sugar, water and cinnamon.

Cook and stir over medium low heat till mixture is slightly thickened and coats a metal spoon (10-12 minutes).

Remove from heat, stir in vanilla and cooked rice.

Turn into a 1-quart casserole.

Beat 1 egg white till soft peaks form.

Gradually add the 1 tablespoon sugar.

Beat till stiff peaks form.

Drop egg mixture in 4 dollops atop pudding.

Bake at 325° till meringue is golden — 12-15 minutes.

Serves 4   each: ½ Meat Exchange
                   1 Bread Exchange

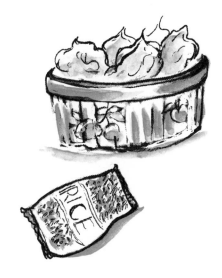

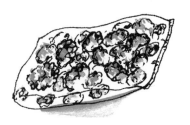

RASPBERRY BAVARIAN CREAM

1 tablespoon unflavored gelatin
2 tablespoons cold water
1 (10-ounce) package frozen raspberries
1 tablespoon orange juice
⅛ teaspoon salt
1 cup evaporated skim milk

Soften gelatin in cold water.

Place over boiling water and stir until dissolved.

Add frozen raspberries, orange juice and salt.

Freeze evaporated milk to a heavy mush.

Beat until stiff and fold raspberry mixture into whipped milk.

Turn into 1 large or 6 individual molds.

Chill until firm.

Serves 6   each: ½ Fruit Exchange
                   ½ Milk Exchange

dessert

154

3D ICE CREAM

Freeze 1 cup skim milk in ice cube trays.
When frozen, place in plastic bag in freezer.
Place one serving of fruit (berries, peaches, applesauce, banana, pineapple) in blender and add frozen milk to make one serving.
Add sweetener, vanilla and cinnamon if desired.
Blend until thick and smooth.

Serves 1   1 Fruit Exchange
                1 Milk Exchange

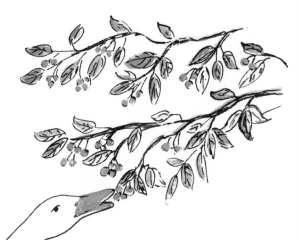

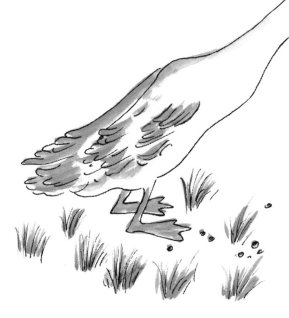

LOW-CALORIE CHEESECAKE

2 tablespoons diet margarine
½ cup graham cracker crumbs
2 cups 2% butterfat cottage cheese
2 tablespoons flour
¼ teaspoon butter-flavored salt
4 eggs, separated
½ cup evaporated skim milk
2 teaspoons vanilla
1 (6-ounce) can frozen orange juice concentrate, defrosted, undiluted

Coat the bottom of a 9-inch spring pan with the diet margarine.
Sprinkle the cracker crumbs over the margarine.
In a bowl whip the cottage cheese, flour and butter-flavored salt until smooth.
Add the egg yolks one at a time, mixing well after each addition.
Stir in the milk, vanilla and orange juice.
In another bowl, beat the egg whites until stiff, and fold them into the cheese batter.
Pour the batter over the crumbs.
Bake in preheated oven at 325° for 1 hour.
Allow it to cool before removing the rim of the pan. Do not invert the cake.

Serves 12   each: 1 Meat Exchange
                         ½ Fruit Exchange

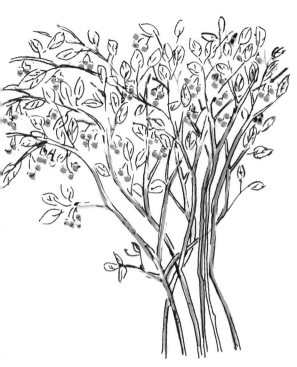

CRANBERRY CHUTNEY

1 bag cranberries — cleaned and washed
½ cup orange juice
2-3 oranges, in segments
½ cup raisins
1 teaspoon cinnamon
1 tablespoon vinegar

Place cranberries and orange juice in pan to boil.
Add oranges, raisins, cinnamon and vinegar.
Bring to a boil and simmer until cranberries pop.

1 tablespoon = 1 Free Exchange

JELLIED BERRY TOPPING

¾ cup ice-cold bottled unsweetened red grape juice
1½ teaspoons unflavored gelatin
1 cup sliced strawberries or raspberries (or other fruit)

Put 2 tablespoons of the grape juice in a small saucepan and sprinkle with the gelatin.
Wait 1 minute, until the gelatin is soft, then heat until the gelatin melts.
Remove from heat and stir in the remaining cold fruit juice.
Refrigerate until syrupy.
Arrange the berries on top of ice cream, pudding or cheesecake; then spoon the gelatin mixture to cover the fruit with a jellied glaze.
Serves 8   each: ½ Fruit Exchange

ORANGE SAUCE

2 oranges
orange juice
¼ cup sugar
2 tablespoons cornstarch
¼ teaspoon salt
1 cup water
2 tablespoons butter or margarine
1 teaspoon lemon juice

Section and chop fruit; drain and reserve juice.
To the reserved juice add additional orange juice to make ½ cup.
In saucepan combine sugar, cornstarch and salt.
Add orange juice and water.
Bring to boiling, reduce heat and simmer 3 minutes, stirring constantly.
Blend in butter, lemon juice and orange pieces.
To be served with Orange French Toast, page 28.

1 tablespoon = ½ Fruit Exchange

dessert

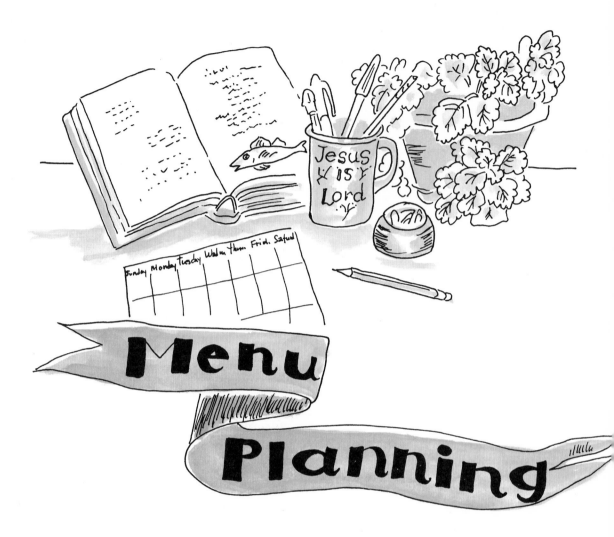

Menu Planning

One of the first things many of us learned in the beginning of 3D was that our families ate the way we felt. If it was a good day, it was a good meal, and if it was a bad day, watch out. The mood of the mother planned the menu of the day — not very spiritual, is it? God has called me and you as Christians to live not according to our feelings but with our commitment to Him first and foremost in our mind.

For most of us, planning our menu was the first step in breaking out of the control we had allowed our feelings to have on the life of our entire family. Instead of cooking the way we felt, we sat down and planned a week's menus, trying very hard to listen to the Lord and to plan according to our family's needs and our financial limitations. I have always firmly recommended that menu planning be done on the day of the week when the ads come out in the local newspaper of all the specials in the grocery stores. At a quiet corner in the house, open the newspaper wide, get your menu planning sheet out of your packet, pour yourself a cup of coffee, ask the Lord to help you, and watch what happens. I promise you that this discipline followed religiously in your house will do more to change your attitude and the attitude of your family in regards to meal time. Unfortunately for many of us, mealtime has never been the blessing that God intended it to be, and a lot of the reason for that has been poor planning and poor organization.

Let me tell you some of the other advantages of menu planning. First, your family can become more a part of meal plans. Your children can participate in the preparing of food for tomorrow by glancing at the menu posted on the refrigerator door. They can set the table properly without asking a dozen questions at the wrong time for you. If the cook gets delayed on a particular day at the church or at the office, the family can be a real blessing by getting things started. Menu planning takes a little more time each week, but it saves a great deal more time in the end. Another good reason for menu planning is that it saves money. You can sit down with those weekly ads and your menus can be planned according to what is being offered on sale at the market. Your grocery list can become absolutely accurate and unnecessary items need not be purchased. Do you know that the grocery store counts on getting you into the store with the ads, but only makes money on what you buy that is not on sale? Attractive, interesting displays sell more items than the consumer imagines. Our eyes are easily satisfied, only to find at the cash register the pain of purchasing that way. With an accurate

grocery list anyone in the family can go shopping. There is no question that your diet will be more carefully followed if your menu is planned ahead. You are able to watch more carefully the types of food you are eating regularly where calories and fats slip in so unnoticed with unplanned meals. Menu planning also prevents more often than not the forgotten food in the freezer. Everyone in the house can think about what needs to come out of the freezer for the next big meal.

Menus for Week 1

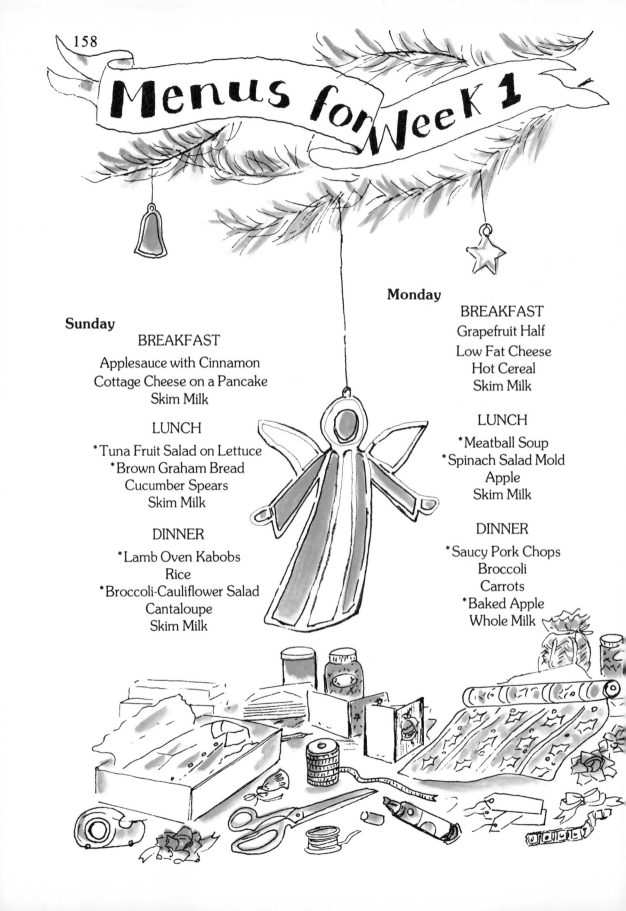

Sunday

BREAKFAST

Applesauce with Cinnamon
Cottage Cheese on a Pancake
Skim Milk

LUNCH

*Tuna Fruit Salad on Lettuce
*Brown Graham Bread
Cucumber Spears
Skim Milk

DINNER

*Lamb Oven Kabobs
Rice
*Broccoli-Cauliflower Salad
Cantaloupe
Skim Milk

Monday

BREAKFAST
Grapefruit Half
Low Fat Cheese
Hot Cereal
Skim Milk

LUNCH

*Meatball Soup
*Spinach Salad Mold
Apple
Skim Milk

DINNER

*Saucy Pork Chops
Broccoli
Carrots
*Baked Apple
Whole Milk

Tuesday

BREAKFAST
Orange
Peanut Butter on Toast
Skim Milk

LUNCH
*Tuna Melt
Green Beans
Carrot Sticks
Skim Milk

DINNER
*Italian Veal Cutlet
*Rice and Mushrooms
Grapefruit Sections with Blueberries
Whole Milk

Wednesday

BREAKFAST
Orange Juice
*Bacon and Cheese Oven Pancakes
Skim Milk

LUNCH
Hamburger on Half Roll
*Stir Fry Vegetables
Tossed Salad
Low-Calorie Dressing
Grapes
Skim Milk

DINNER
*Oven Poached Haddock
*Tangy Potato Salad
Beets
*Spinach Bake
*Apple Salad

Thursday

BREAKFAST
Orange Juice
Poached Egg
English Muffin Half with Butter
Whole Milk

LUNCH
*Carrot Souffle
Leftover *Tangy Potato Salad
Banana Half
Skim Milk

DINNER
*Chicken-Vegetable Stir Fry
Rice
*Lemon Carrots
Mandarin Oranges/Banana Slices
sprinkled with Coconut
Skim Milk

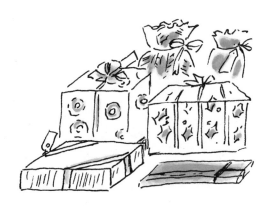

Friday

BREAKFAST

Low-Calorie Cranberry Juice
Cottage Cheese Broiled on Muffin Half
Whole Milk

LUNCH

*Fresh Mushroom-Cheese Pie
*Glazed Turnips
Fresh Strawberries
Skim Milk

DINNER

Low-Calorie Cranberry Juice
Ham Slices
*Potato Bread
Raw Vegetable Platter
*Cheesy Bean Casserole
*Two-Tone Molded Dessert

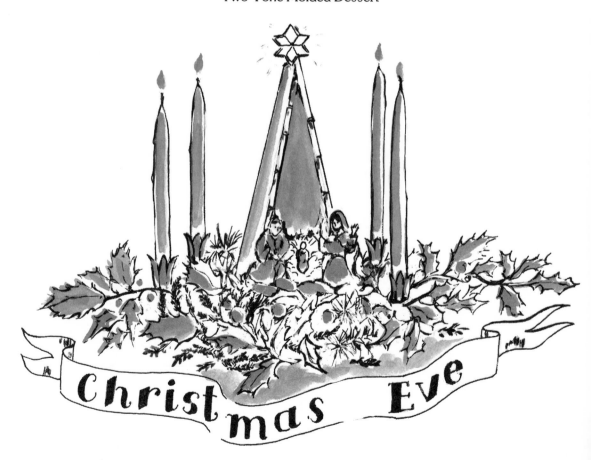

Christmas Eve

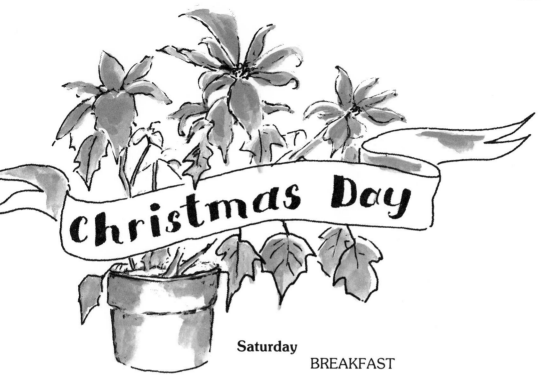

Christmas Day

Saturday

BREAKFAST

Orange Juice
Scrambled Eggs
Christmas Bread
Whole Milk

LUNCH

*Jellied Chicken Loaf on Lettuce
Corn Muffin
Broccoli
Carrot and Celery Sticks
Skim Milk

DINNER

Roast Prime Rib
Baked Potato with Sour Cream
*Spinach Loaf
Green Beans with Mushrooms
*Frozen Pineapple Dessert

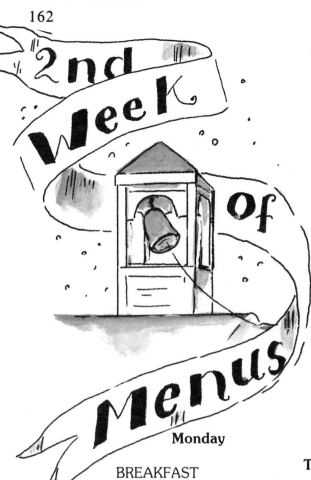

2nd Week of Menus

Sunday

BREAKFAST

Grapefruit Half
Fried Egg
Toast with Butter
Skim Milk

LUNCH

*French Onion Soup
*Crab Salad
Orange
Skim Milk

DINNER

*Stir Fry Beef with Broccoli
Rice
*Spinach Salad
Hard Boiled Egg
*True Fruit Salad
Skim Milk

Monday

BREAKFAST

Fresh Fruit
Low Fat Cottage Cheese
Bran Muffin with Butter
Skim Milk

LUNCH

*Polynesian Sandwich
Tossed Salad
Low-Calorie Dressing
Skim Milk

DINNER

*Round-Up Pork Chops
Small Potato
*Broccoli-Cauliflower Salad
*Apple Compote
Skim Milk

Tuesday

BREAKFAST

Grapefruit Half
Peanut Butter on Toast
Skim Milk

LUNCH

*Cottage Cheese Delight Dressing on
Vegetable and Fruit Platter
Hot Roll
Skim Milk

DINNER

*Stuffed Pepper
Lettuce-Radish Salad
French Dressing
*Hawaiian Ice
Skim Milk

Wednesday

BREAKFAST

Orange Juice
Hard Boiled Egg
Toast with Butter
Skim Milk

LUNCH

*Cream of Tomato Soup
Broiled Hamburger
Bagel Half
Sliced Tomato and Cucumber
Peach

DINNER

*Diet Lasagna
Italian Bread
Tossed Salad with
Vinegar Dressing
Fresh Fruit Cup
Skim Milk

Thursday

BREAKFAST

Cottage Cheese
Raisin Bran Cereal
Whole Milk

LUNCH

*Cheese Frank Sandwich
Green Pepper Strips
Celery Sticks
Pineapple Chunks
Skim Milk

DINNER

*Breaded Liver with Onions
Spinach
*Baked Butternut Squash with Butter
Sliced Bananas
Whole Milk

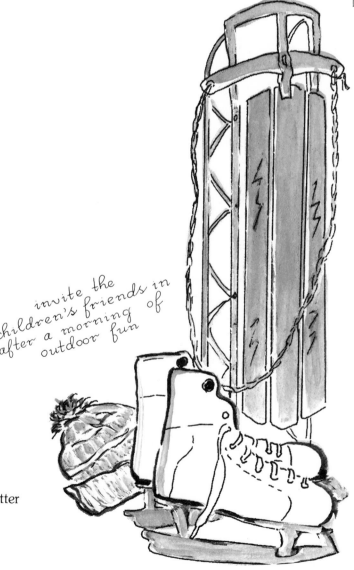

invite the children's friends in after a morning of outdoor fun

BREAKFAST
Stewed Prunes
Soft Boiled Egg
Wheat Toast with Butter
Whole Milk

LUNCH
Cold Beef Slices
Whole Wheat Roll
Carrot and Celery Sticks
*Fresh Fruit Melon Compote
Milk

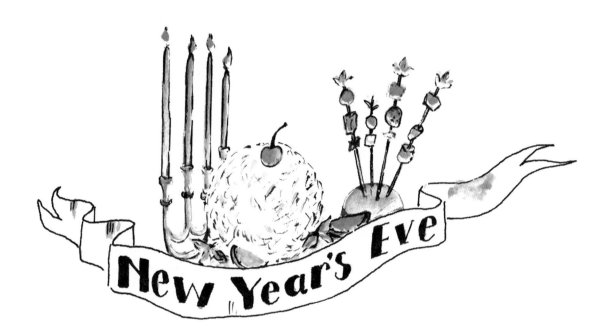

New Year's Eve

DINNER

Assorted Appetizers:
  Raw Vegetables with Dip
  Cheese and Crackers
  Fondue
  Herbed Mushrooms

Hot and Cold Punches:
  *Mint Berry Splash
  Hot Apple Cider

*Chicken Cordon Bleu
Fresh Steamed, Seasoned Broccoli,
Cauliflower and Carrot Medley
*Spinach Salad with Bacon
Oven Roasted Potatoes
*Snowball Cake

166

Menus for the 3rd Week

Sunday

BREAKFAST

Orange Juice
English Muffin Half with Butter
Poached Egg
Skim Milk

LUNCH

Open Faced Chicken Sandwich
*Lemon Carrots
Green Pepper Strips
Apple
Skim Milk

DINNER

*Tamale Pie
Tossed Salad with Cheddar Cheese
*Pineapple Vinegar Dressing
*Fruit Salad
Skim Milk

Monday

BREAKFAST

*Orange French Toast
*Orange Sauce
Skim Milk

LUNCH

*Easy Vegetable Soup
Cheese and Crackers
Fresh Fruit
Skim Milk

DINNER

*Meal-in-One Casserole
Green Salad
Low-Calorie Dressing
Fresh Fruit and Cheese Platter
Skim Milk

Tuesday

BREAKFAST

Orange Juice
Toast with Butter
Cottage Cheese
Skim Milk

LUNCH

*Chicken-Apple Salad on Lettuce
Whole Wheat Bread with Butter
Tomato Slices
Cucumber Sticks
Skim Milk
*(Use chicken in place of turkey in
Turkey-Apple Salad recipe)

DINNER

*Harvest Pork Chops
Baked Acorn Squash
Broccoli
*Applesauce Dessert
Whole Milk

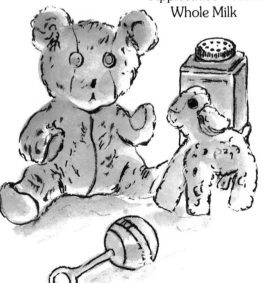

Wednesday
BREAKFAST
Grapefruit Half
Soft Boiled Egg
Bacon
Toast
Skim Milk

LUNCH
Hot Tomato Juice
Fresh Fruit Plate (Watermelon, Canteloupe,
Strawberries, Pineapple and Green
Grapes)
Scoop of Cottage Cheese
Brown Graham Bread

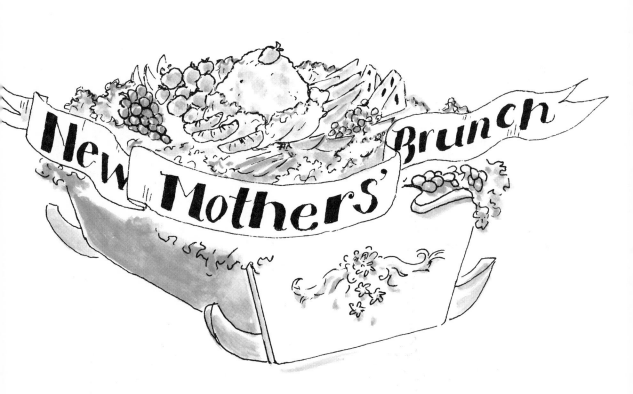

DINNER
*Applesauce Meat Loaf
*Cauliflower Italiano
*Carrot-Raisin Salad
Whole Milk

Thursday

BREAKFAST

*Overnight French Toast
with Fruit
Bacon
Skim Milk

LUNCH

*Salmon Salad
Chef Salad with Croutons
Low-Calorie Dressing
Fresh Pear
Skim Milk

DINNER

*Pot o' Gold Chicken
Tossed Salad
Low-Calorie Dressing
Broiled Tomato
Skim Milk

Friday

BREAKFAST

Orange Juice
Pam-fried Egg
Wheat Toast with Butter
Skim Milk

LUNCH

*Fresh Mushroom-Cheese Pie
Green Beans
Orange
Skim Milk

DINNER

*Curried Chicken on Rice
Broccoli
*Low-Calorie Cheesecake with
*Jellied Berry Topping
Whole Milk

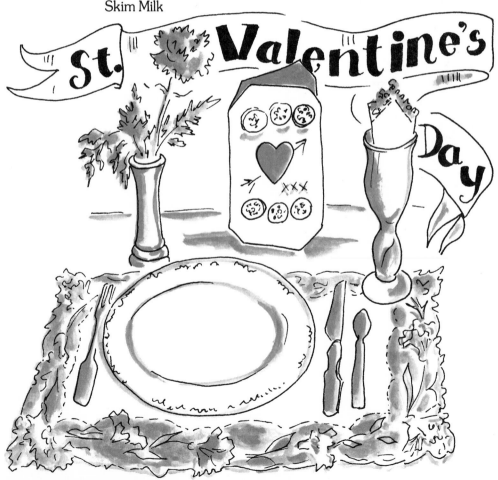

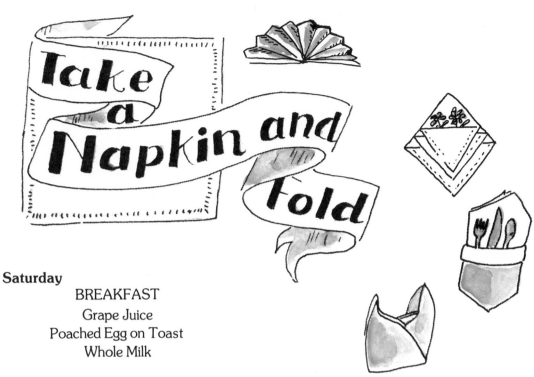

Saturday

BREAKFAST
Grape Juice
Poached Egg on Toast
Whole Milk

LUNCH
Cheddar Cheese and Crackers
*Zesty Tomato-Cabbage Soup
Raw Broccoli and Cauliflower
Orange
Skim Milk

DINNER
*Fresh Fish
*Parsley Carrots and Potatoes
Broccoli
*True Fruit Salad
Skim Milk

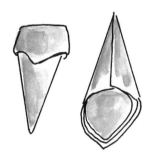

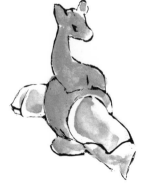

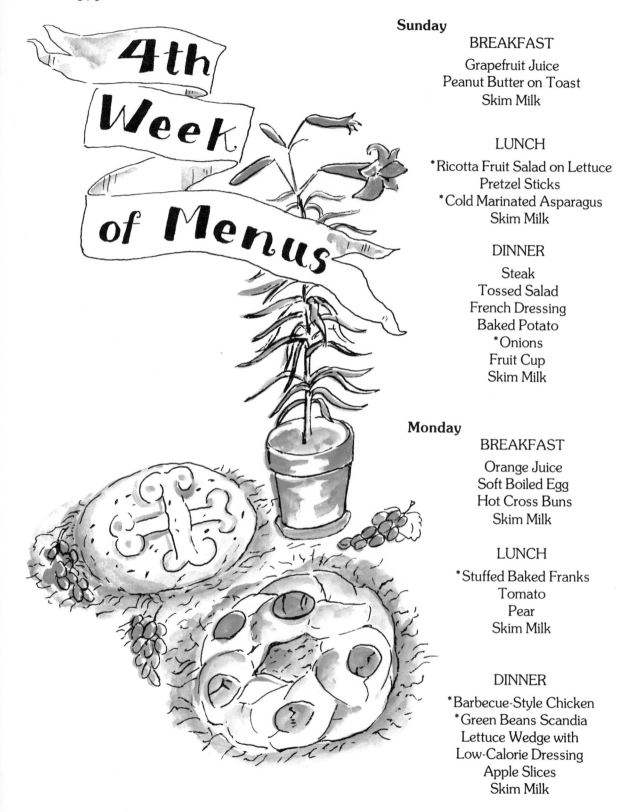

4th Week of Menus

Sunday

BREAKFAST
Grapefruit Juice
Peanut Butter on Toast
Skim Milk

LUNCH
*Ricotta Fruit Salad on Lettuce
Pretzel Sticks
*Cold Marinated Asparagus
Skim Milk

DINNER
Steak
Tossed Salad
French Dressing
Baked Potato
*Onions
Fruit Cup
Skim Milk

Monday

BREAKFAST
Orange Juice
Soft Boiled Egg
Hot Cross Buns
Skim Milk

LUNCH
*Stuffed Baked Franks
Tomato
Pear
Skim Milk

DINNER
*Barbecue-Style Chicken
*Green Beans Scandia
Lettuce Wedge with
Low-Calorie Dressing
Apple Slices
Skim Milk

menus

Tuesday

BREAKFAST
Orange Juice
*Bacon Cheese Oven Pancake
Skim Milk

LUNCH
Cottage Cheese
*Canadian Green Beans
*Rye Roll with Butter
Applesauce
Skim Milk

DINNER
Baked Ham
Mashed Potato
*Baked Spiced Squash
Tomato Slices
Pineapple Ring

Wednesday

BREAKFAST
Pineapple Juice
Poached Egg
Wheat Toast
Whole Milk

LUNCH
Open-Faced Cheese and
Tomato Sandwich
Carrot and Celery Sticks
*Ambrosia Shake

DINNER
*Baked Turbot in Tomato Juice
*Stuffed Idaho Potato
*Layered Vegetable Salad
*Orange Cranberry Cooler

Holy Week

Almighty God, whose most dear Son went not up to joy but first he suffered pain, and entered not into glory before he was crucified: Mercifully grant that we, walking in the way of the cross, may find it none other than the way of life and peace; through the same thy Son Jesus Christ our Lord. Amen.

*Monday before Easter Collect
from the Book of Common Prayer*

172

Thursday

BREAKFAST

Pancake with Sliced Peaches
Cheddar Cheese
Whole Milk

LUNCH

*June Soup
Tossed Salad with Egg and Ham
*Pineapple-Vinegar Dressing
Rye Roll
Apple
Skim Milk

Maundy Thursday

DINNER

Roasted Shank Bone of lamb — represents the sacrifice

Hard Boiled Egg — sliced and served and can be dipped in salt water to represent tears and mourning over the destruction of the temple

Bitter Herbs — horseradish root, ground horseradish and endive or lettuce — represents suffering but also life

Mixture of chopped apples, nuts, raisins and cinnamon — symbolizes red clay of Egypt which the children of Israel used when they were forced to make bricks for Pharaoh

Unleavened Bread — as told to Moses to prepare for swift departure from Egypt

Friday

BREAKFAST

Orange Juice
Scrambled Egg
Hot Cross Bun
Skim Milk

LUNCH

*Hamburger Stuffed Rolls
Sauteed Mushrooms
Sliced Tomatoes
*Baked Apple
Skim Milk

DINNER

*Fish Chowder
Chef Salad
French Dressing
Melon Balls

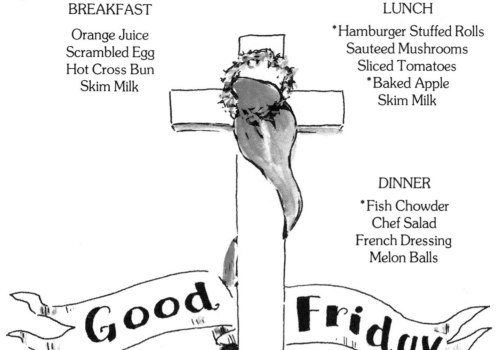

Saturday

BREAKFAST

Grapefruit Half
Melted Cheese on
English Muffin Half
Whole Milk

LUNCH

*Crab Salad
Small Dinner Roll with Butter
Lettuce and Tomato Slices
Apple
Skim Milk

DINNER

*Hungarian Skillet Ragout
Tossed Salad
Italian Dressing
Molded Pineapple Salad
*Rice Meringue Pudding

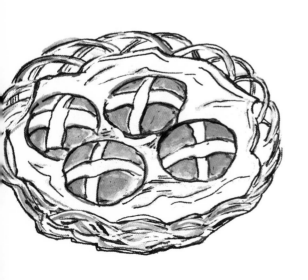

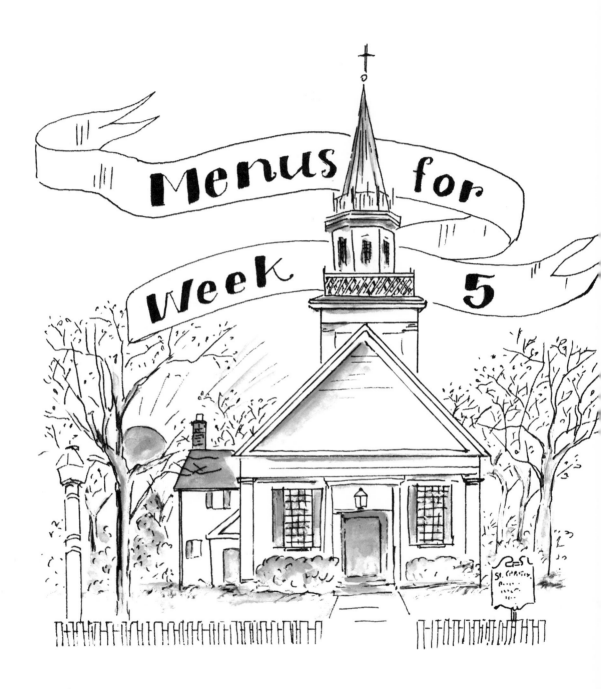

Menus for Week 5

BREAKFAST

Orange Juice
Baked Eggs
Canadian Bacon
Assorted Breads

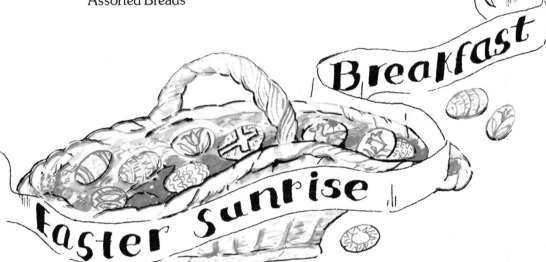

LUNCH

Hard-Cooked Eggs
*Spinach Salad with Bacon
Low-Calorie Italian Dressing
Melba Toast
Apple
Skim Milk

DINNER

*Chicken Cordon Bleu
Asparagus
*Cabbage Medley
*Peach Parfait
Whole Milk

Monday

BREAKFAST

Stewed Prunes
Poached Egg
Whole Wheat Toast
Skim Milk

LUNCH

Open-Faced Ham and Cheese
Sandwich on Rye
Dill Pickles
Lettuce and Tomato Salad
Low-Calorie Dressing
Canned Peach Half
Skim Milk

DINNER

*Oven Beef Stew
*Johnny Cake
Lettuce Wedge
*Two-Tone Molded Dessert
Skim Milk

Tuesday

BREAKFAST

Orange Juice
Cottage Cheese
Cinnamon-Raisin English Muffin Ha
Whole Milk

LUNCH

*Cheese Frank Sandwich
Carrot Sticks
*Spicy Cole Slaw
Apple Skim Milk

DINNER

*Flounder Continental
*Perfection Salad
Green Peas
*Low-Calorie Cheesecake
with Strawberries

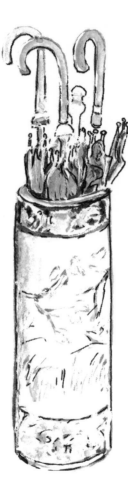

Wednesday

BREAKFAST

Low-Calorie Cranberry Juice
Pam-fried Egg
Toast with Butter
Skim Milk

LUNCH

*Swiss Cheese Hawaiian
Whole Wheat Saltines
Celery
Radishes
Skim Milk

DINNER

*Baked Marinated Chicken
*Potatoes Au Gratin
Broccoli
*Carrot Raisin Salad

Thursday

BREAKFAST

*Orange French Toast with
*Orange Sauce
Bacon
Skim Milk

LUNCH

*Polynesian Sandwich
*Spinach Salad with Fruit
Celery
Orange

DINNER

*Diet Lasagna
French Bread
Green Salad
Low-Calorie Dressing
*3D Ice Cream

Friday

BREAKFAST

Apricots
Herbed Scrambled Egg
English Muffin Half with Butter
Skim Milk

LUNCH

Ham Slice
Cheesy Bean Casserole
Dill Pickle
Cherry Tomatoes
Orange
Skim Milk

DINNER

Baked Pork Chop with Apple Slices
Butternut Squash
*French Almond Green Beans
Whole Milk

Saturday

BREAKFAST

Orange Juice
Cheese Slice
Cold Cereal
Whole Milk

LUNCH

*Souffle Tuna Aspic
Rye Wafer
Hot Green Beans
Melon Wedge
Whole Milk

DINNER

*Breaded Liver
Noodles with Butter
*Brussels Sprouts in Mushroom Sauce
Carrots
Melon Balls

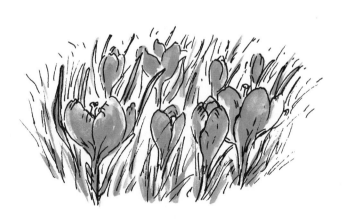

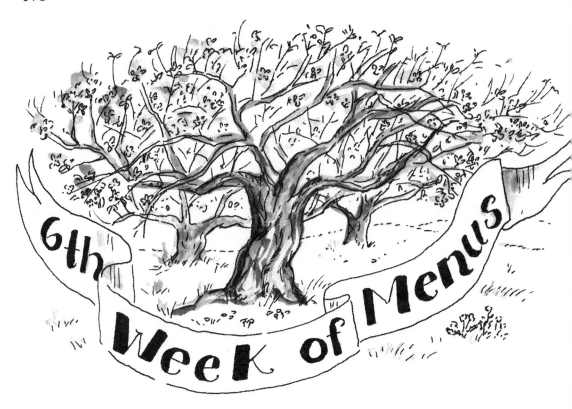

6th Week of Menus

Sunday

BREAKFAST

Sliced Strawberries
Cottage Cheese on Toast
Skim Milk

LUNCH

*Open Faced Hot Dog Reubens
Cherry Tomatoes
Fruit Cup
Skim Milk

DINNER

Turkey with *Apple Bacon Stuffing
Broccoli-Carrot-Cauliflower Medley
*Cranberry Chutney
*Low-Calorie Cheesecake
Skim Milk

Monday

BREAKFAST

Grapefruit Half
3-Minute Egg
Toast with Butter
Skim Milk

LUNCH

*Ham Stuffed Rolls
Green Beans
Fresh Fruit
Skim Milk

DINNER

*Beef-Cabbage Casserole
Buttered Boiled Potato
Sliced Banana and Blueberries
Skim Milk

Tuesday

BREAKFAST

Blueberries
Cheddar Cheese
Cereal
Skim Milk

LUNCH

Broiled Hamburger on
English Muffin Half
Sliced Onion
Sauteed Mushrooms
*Baked Apple
Skim Milk

DINNER

Warm Turkey Slices
Sweet Potato
*Chinese Asparagus
*Citrus Winter Salad
Skim Milk

Wednesday

BREAKFAST

Apple Juice
Broiled Muenster Cheese
on Rye Toast
Skim Milk

LUNCH

*Tuna Fruit Salad
Small Roll
Spinach
Skim Milk

DINNER

*Pot Roast Supreme
Potatoes and Carrots
Green Beans with Mushrooms
*Peach Parfait
Whole Milk

Thursday

BREAKFAST

Oatmeal with Raisins
Wedge of Cheese
Skim Milk

LUNCH

*June's Soup
Cheese and Crackers
*Banana Milkshake

DINNER

*Quick Lamb
*Layered Vegetable Salad
*Peach Parfait
Skim Milk

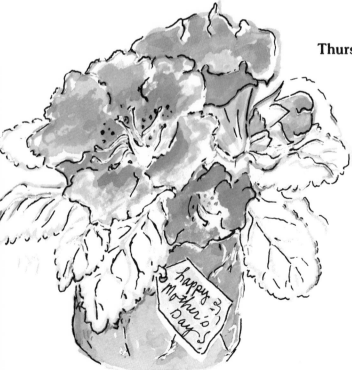

Friday

BREAKFAST

Orange Juice
Scrambled Egg
Roll with Butter
Whole Milk

LUNCH

*Mushroom Asparagus Omelet
Carrots
Celery
Fresh Strawberries
Skim Milk

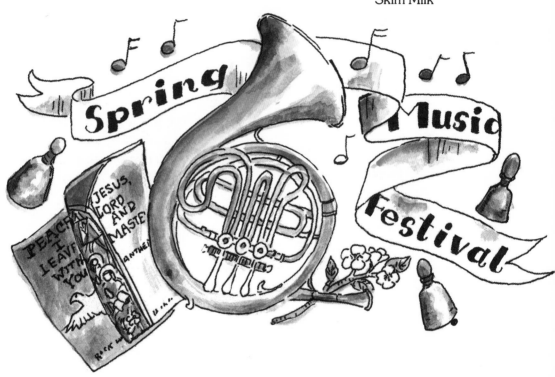

DINNER

*Diet Cabbage Lasagna
Italian Bread
Tossed Salad
Low Calorie Italian Dressing
Fruit Cup

Saturday

BREAKFAST

Melon Wedge
*Overnight French Toast
Bacon
Skim Milk

LUNCH

*Ham Stuffed Roll
Carrots/Celery Sticks
Dill Pickle
Fresh Strawberries
Skim Milk

DINNER

*Fish Roll-Ups
Potato
*Marinated Vegetable Medley
*Frozen Fruit Dessert

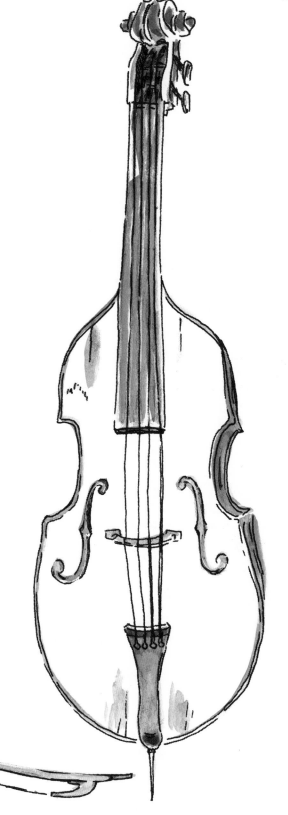

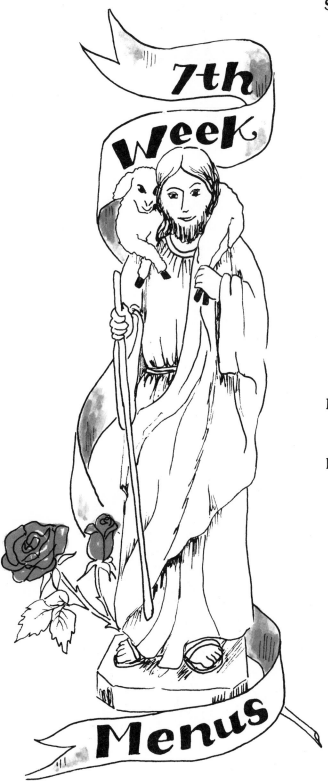

7th Week Menus

Sunday

BREAKFAST

Orange Juice
*Apple Whole Wheat Pancakes
Ham

LUNCH

*Spinach Quiche
Vegetable Relish Tray
*Berry Shake

DINNER

*Oven Steak Dinner
Lettuce Wedge
Low-Calorie Dressing
*True Fruit Salad
Skim Milk

Monday

BREAKFAST

Applesauce
Broiled Muenster Cheese on Rye Toast
Skim Milk

LUNCH

Sliced Chicken
Corn Muffin
*Marinated Asparagus
Celery Stalks
Apple
Skim Milk

DINNER

*Applesauce Meatloaf
*Spinach Salad with Fruit
Celery and Carrot Sticks

Wednesday

BREAKFAST

Oatmeal with Raisins
Wedge of Cheese
Whole Milk

Tuesday

BREAKFAST

Grapefruit Half
3-Minute Egg
Toast with Butter
Skim Milk

LUNCH

Chef Salad with Sliced Ham
Hard-cooked Egg
Low-Calorie Italian Dressing
*Brown Graham Bread
Orange
Skim Milk

LUNCH

Left-over *Applesauce Meatloaf
Stewed Tomatoes
Carrot and Celery Sticks
Sliced Peaches
Skim Milk

DINNER

*Pineapple Perch Fillets
Boiled Potato with Butter
*Pickled Beets
*Scalloped Spinach
*Apple Salad

DINNER

*Quick Lamb
Cauliflower
Tossed Salad
*Low-Calorie Ranch Dressing
*Mint-Berry Splash

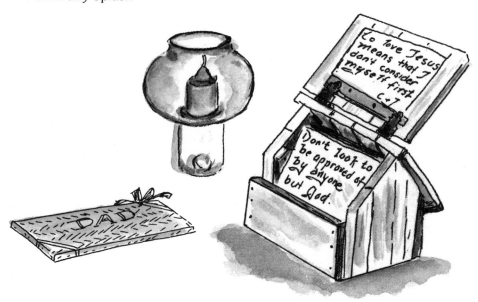

Thursday

BREAKFAST

Sliced Strawberries
Cottage Cheese on Toast
Whole Milk

LUNCH

*Open Face Hot Dog Reuben
Carrot Sticks
Fruit Salad
Skim Milk

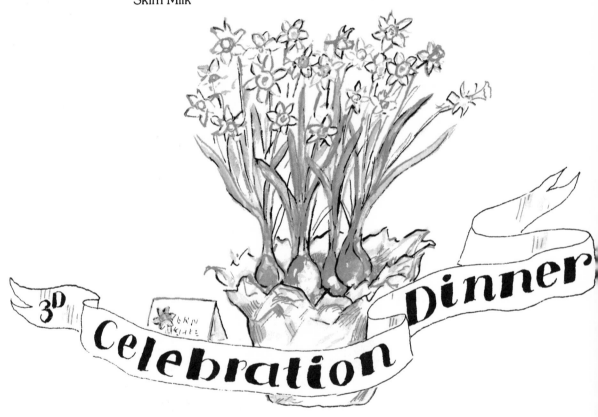

3D Celebration Dinner

V-8 Juice
Crackers
*Fish Roll-Ups with Broccoli Bud Garnish
*Spicy Cole Slaw
*Rye and Whole Wheat Rolls
*Frozen Pineapple Dessert

Cranberry Juice and Soda
Vegetable and Fruit Platter
*Chicken Crepes Elegante
*Lemon Carrots
*Green Salad Vinaigrette
Rolls
*Peach Parfait

Friday

BREAKFAST

Orange Juice
Scrambled Egg
Toast with Butter
Skim Milk

LUNCH

*Mushroom Asparagus Omelet
Holland Rusks
Sliced Tomatoes
Orange and Grapefruit Sections
Skim Milk

DINNER

White Grape Juice and Soda Water
*Chicken Chow Mein
Spinach and Mushroom Salad
Italian Dressing
Whole Milk

Saturday

BREAKFAST

Melon Wedge
French Toast with Butter
Bacon
Skim Milk

LUNCH

*Vegetable Soup
Wedges of Apple and Cheese
Skim Milk

DINNER

*Spanish Pork Chops
*Company Beets
Asparagus Spears
*Rice Meringue Pudding
Skim Milk

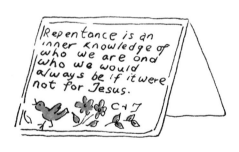

Repentance is an inner knowledge of who we are and who we would always be if it were not for Jesus.

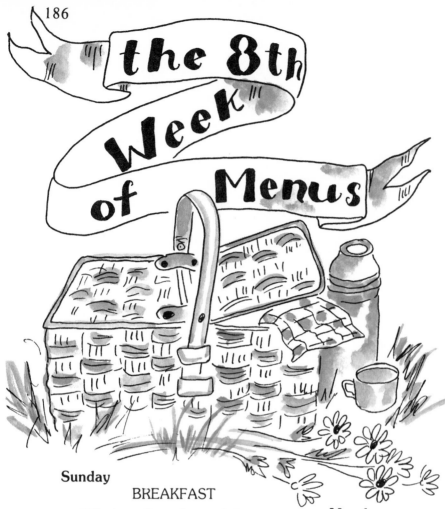

the 8th Week of Menus

Sunday

BREAKFAST
*Blueberry Pancakes with Butter
Cottage Cheese

LUNCH
*Zesty Tomato-Cabbage Soup
Cheese Spread on
Rye Crisp Crackers
Pineapple
Skim Milk

DINNER
*Veal Marengo
Green Beans Almondine
Tossed Salad
Low-Calorie Dressing
Small Crusty Roll with Butter
*Frozen Fruit Dessert

Monday

BREAKFAST
Orange Juice
Boiled Egg
Toast with Butter
Skim Milk

LUNCH
*Shrimp and Tuna Bake
Cucumber in Sour Cream
Fresh Pineapple and Blueberries
Skim Milk

DINNER
*Zucchini Beef Boats
*Whole Wheat Bran Muffins
*Orange Milkshake

Tuesday

BREAKFAST

Banana Half
Melted Cheese on Toast
Bacon
Skim Milk

LUNCH

*Orange Baked Chicken
*Green Salad Vinaigrette
Raw Vegetable Platter with Dip
Angel Food Cake
with Strawberries and Blueberries
Low Calorie Ice Tea

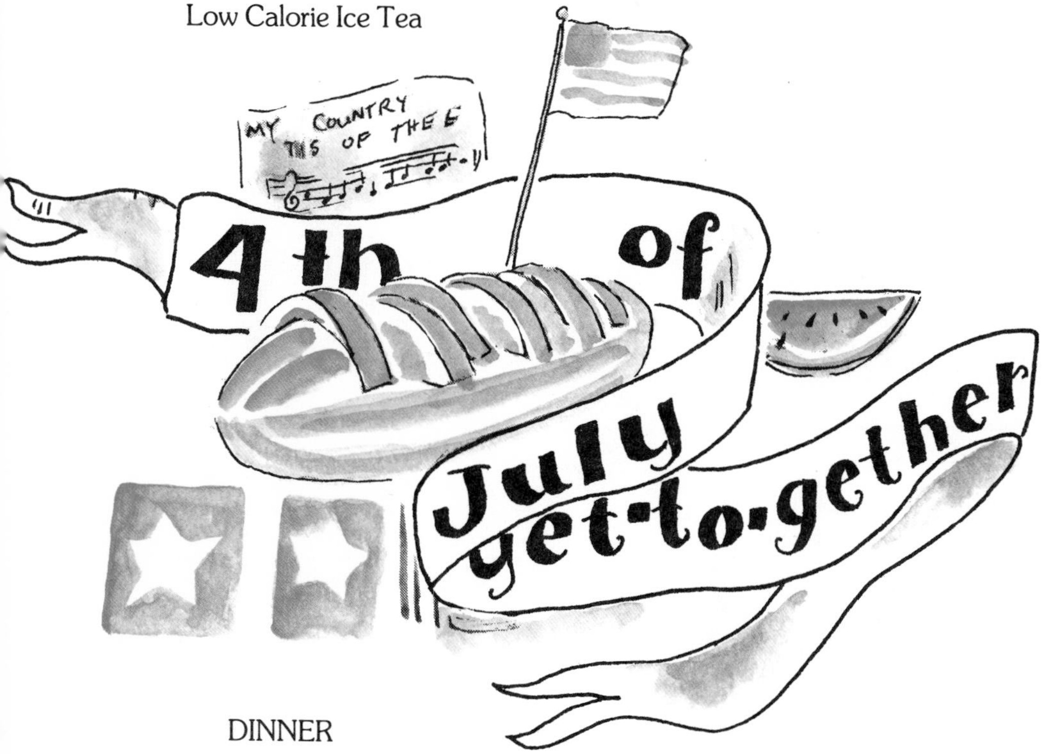

4th of July get-to-gether

MY COUNTRY TIS OF THEE

DINNER

*Stuffed Flank Steak
Summer Squash
*Creole Eggplant
Watermelon
Whole Milk

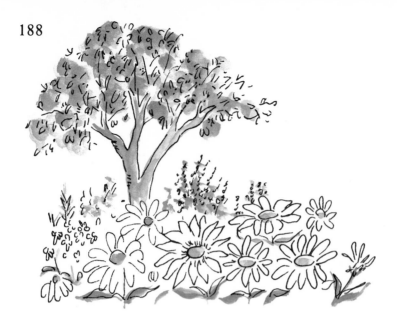

Wednesday

BREAKFAST

Plain Yogurt
with Sliced Bananas
Poached Egg
Toast

LUNCH

*Chicken Potato Salad
*Skillet Zucchini
Tomato Slices
Broiled Grapefruit Half
Skim Milk

DINNER

*Shish Kabobs
Rice
Brussels Sprouts
*Lime-Melon Mold
Whole Milk

Thursday

BREAKFAST

*Breakfast Cobbler
Coffee

LUNCH

*Cheese Omelette
with Chicken
Toasted English Muffin
Asparagus Spears
Cucumber Sticks
*Molded Pineapple Salad
Skim Milk

DINNER

*Baked Fish
Peas with Pearl Onions
*Zucchini with Garlic
*Frozen Pineapple Dessert

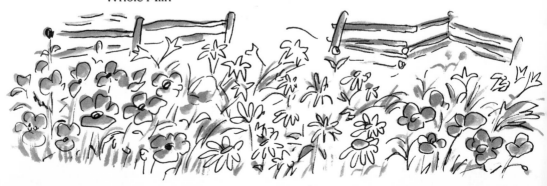

Saturday

BREAKFAST
Strawberries
Broiled Cottage Cheese on Toast
Whole Milk

LUNCH
*Reuben Sandwich
Tossed Salad
Low-Calorie Dressing
Cantaloupe Wedge
Skim Milk

DINNER
*Curried Chicken on Rice
Peas with Mushrooms
Lettuce Wedge
Low-Calorie Dressing
*Hawaiian Ice
Skim Milk

Friday

BREAKFAST
Grapefruit Juice
Cube Cheddar Cheese
*Lower-Calorie Granola
Skim Milk

LUNCH
Ham Slice
*Cheese-Broccoli Bake
Tomato Wedge
Apricots
Skim Milk

DINNER
*Sesame Liver Sauté with Onions
Broccoli
Mashed Potato with Butter
*Fresh Fruit Compote
Whole Milk

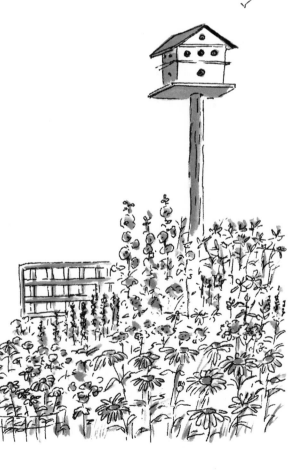

190

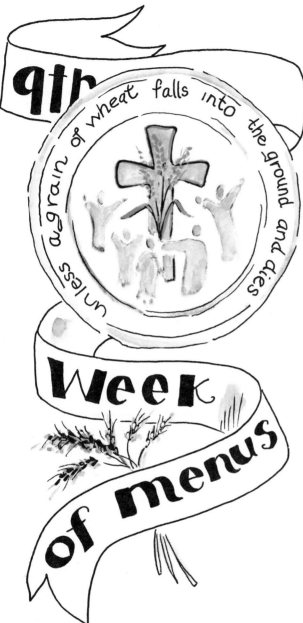

Sunday

BREAKFAST
Grapefruit Half
Poached Egg
Toast
Whole Milk

LUNCH
*Broccoli Timbales
Cheese Slice
Rye Bread with Butter
Tomato Juice
Pineapple Chunks
Skim Milk

DINNER
Turkey with Vegetable Stuffing
*Cranberry Bread
*Tomato Zucchini Casserole
*Lime Melon Mold
Skim Milk

Monday

BREAKFAST
Orange Juice
Cottage Cheese
Bacon
Wheat Toast
Skim Milk

LUNCH
*Turkey and Apple Salad
*Rye Roll with Butter
Carrots
*Cabbage in Bacon
Skim Milk

DINNER
*Hungarian Skillet Ragout
Green Salad
Italian Dressing
*Peach Pie
Skim Milk

Tuesday

BREAKFAST

Grapefruit Juice
*Cheese Omelet
Bran Muffin
Skim Milk

ORANGE CUPS

Cut top off an orange in a scalloped design.
Scoop out pulp and mix with 2 tablespoons
crushed pineapple. Return ½ cup of fruit
mixture to orange cup. Top with diet
whipped topping.

Each Orange cup: 1 Fruit Exchange

LUNCH

*Zesty Tomato Cabbage Soup
*Ham Stuffed Rolls
*Broccoli-Cauliflower Salad
Orange Cups

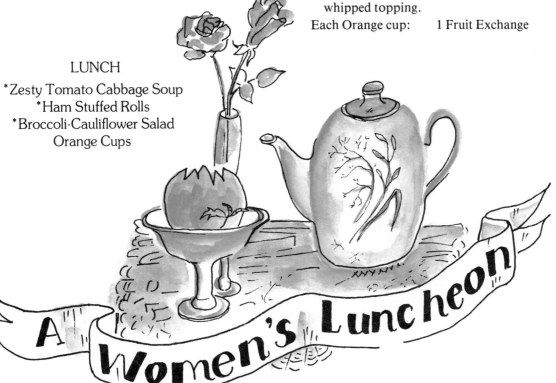

A Women's Luncheon

DINNER

*Zucchini Beef Boats
Cottage Cheese
Dinner Roll
*Strawberry Sponge
Skim Milk

Wednesday

BREAKFAST

Orange Slices
Peanut Butter on Toast
Skim Milk

LUNCH

*Turkey and Apple Salad
on Lettuce
Wheat Crackers
Buttered Broccoli
Skim Milk

DINNER

*Lemon Whitefish Bake
Baked Potato with Butter
*Beets and Beet Tops
Cole Slaw
*Lemon-Orange Gelatin
Skim Milk

Thursday

BREAKFAST

Grapefruit Half
Cheddar Cheese
*Lower-Calorie Granola
Skim Milk

LUNCH

Tomato Stuffed with
*Tuna Salad
Banana Half
Skim Milk

DINNER

Broiled Sirloin Steak
*Grated Potato and Turnip Salad
Sliced Fresh Tomatoes
*Sunshine Zap
Whole Milk

Friday

BREAKFAST

Strawberries
*Baked French Toast with Butter
Whole Milk

LUNCH

*Green and Red Pepper Casserole
Whole Wheat Roll with Butter
Summer Squash
Banana Half
Skim Milk

DINNER

*Sesame Liver Saute with Onions
*Summer Squash
*Lemon-Orange Gelatin
Whole Milk

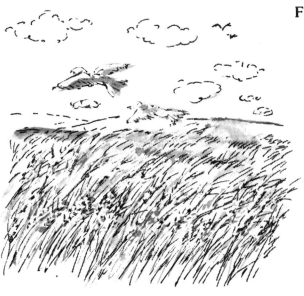

Saturday

BREAKFAST

Orange
*Breakfast Custard Pudding
Bacon

LUNCH

Cheese
*Zesty Tomato Cabbage Soup
Wheat Bread Stick
Blueberries
Whole Milk

DINNER

Baked Ham
Mashed Potatoes with Butter
*Green Beans Provencale
Tomato Slices
*Baked Crimson Pears
Skim Milk

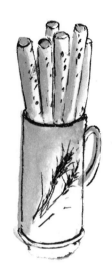

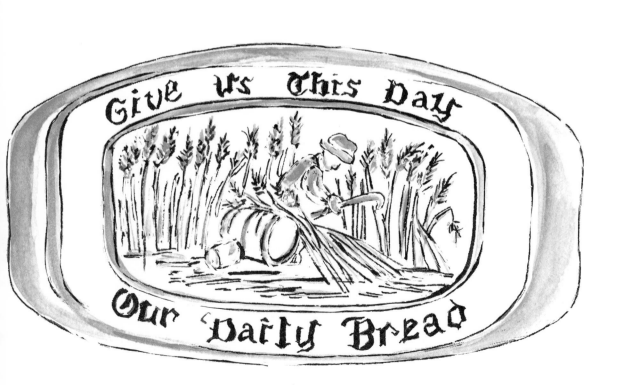

Give Us This Day Our Daily Bread

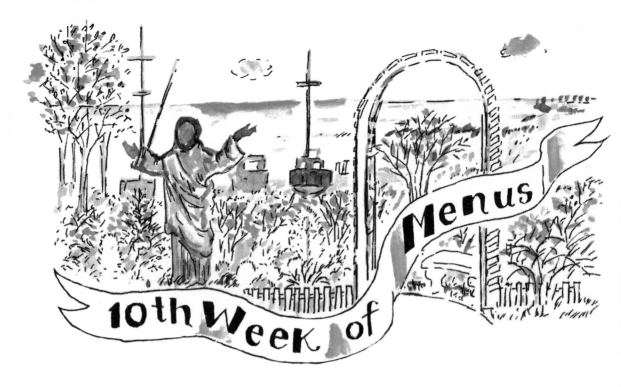

10th Week of Menus

Sunday

BREAKFAST

Orange Juice
Scrambled Egg
Corn Muffin
Skim Milk

LUNCH

Penny Sliced Hot Dogs in
*Cream of Celery Soup
Tossed Salad
Low-Calorie Dressing
Apple Sections

DINNER

*Baked Turbot in Tomato Juice
Roll
*Spinach Salad with Hot Sauce
*Pineapple Slush

Monday

BREAKFAST

Fresh Sliced Peaches
Cottage Cheese on English Muffin Half
Whole Milk

LUNCH

*Chicken and Potato Salad
*Skillet Zucchini
Sliced Tomatoes
Fresh Fruit
Skim Milk

DINNER

*Chicken Livers on Toast
Broccoli Spears
*Pickled Beets
Orange Sections
Whole Milk

Tuesday

BREAKFAST

Grapefruit Juice
*Baked Egg on Whole Wheat Toast
Skim Milk

LUNCH

*Zucchini and Tomato Omelet
*Fruit Float
Skim Milk

DINNER

*Baked Salmon Loaf
Peas
*Marinated Vegetable Medley
Grapes

Thursday

BREAKFAST

Banana Half
Cheese Melted on English Muffin Half
Skim Milk

LUNCH

*Cheese Broccoli Bake
Tossed Salad
*Cottage Cheese Delight Dressing
Apple
Skim Milk

DINNER

*Mushroom Cocktail
Veal Cutlets
Baked Potato with Sour Cream
Green and Wax Beans
Grapefruit Half
Whole Milk

Wednesday

BREAKFAST

Hot Applesauce
*Baked French Toast
Low-Calorie Hot Chocolate

LUNCH

*Salmon Croquettes
Whole Wheat Bread with Butter
Broccoli
Tomato Slices
Peaches
Skim Milk

DINNER

*Chicken in a Crock Pot
Rice with Butter
Green Beans
*Orange-Dilled Carrots
Peach Parfait
Whole Milk

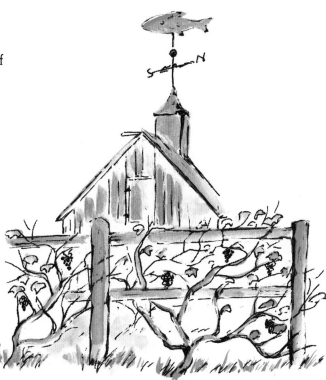

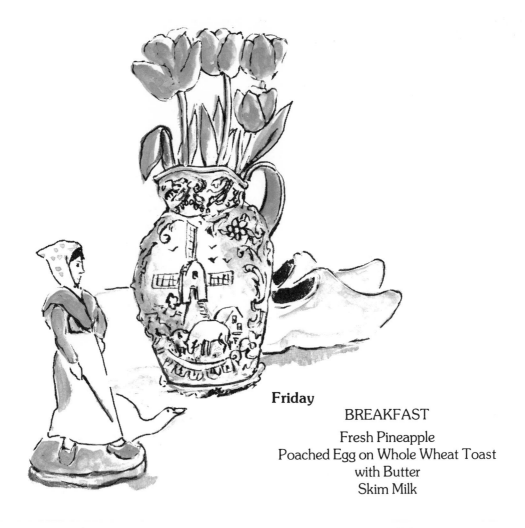

Friday

BREAKFAST

Fresh Pineapple
Poached Egg on Whole Wheat Toast
with Butter
Skim Milk

LUNCH

*Tuna Melt
*Romanian Vegetable Potpourri
Tomato Slices
Skim Milk

DINNER

*Dutch Beef Almondine
Long Grain Rice
Green Beans
Sliced Peaches
Skim Milk

Saturday

BREAKFAST

Orange Juice
*Cottage Cheese Filled Crepe
Whole Milk

LUNCH

Cold Sliced Chicken
*Gazpacho
Broccoli
Sliced Peaches
Skim Milk

*Moo Goo Gai Pan
Long Grain Rice
*Chinese Asparagus
*Molded Pineapple Salad
Lemon Sherbet

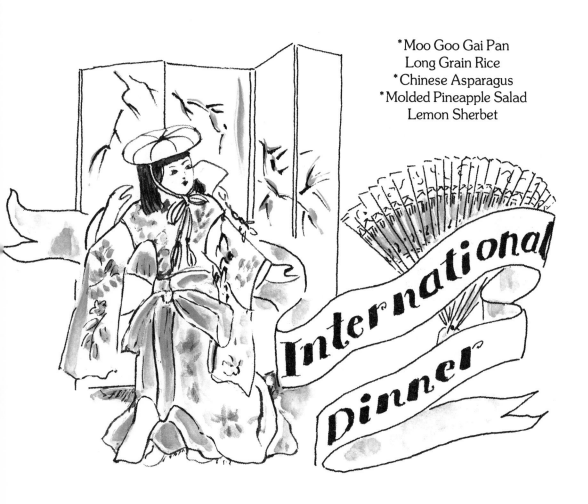

International Dinner

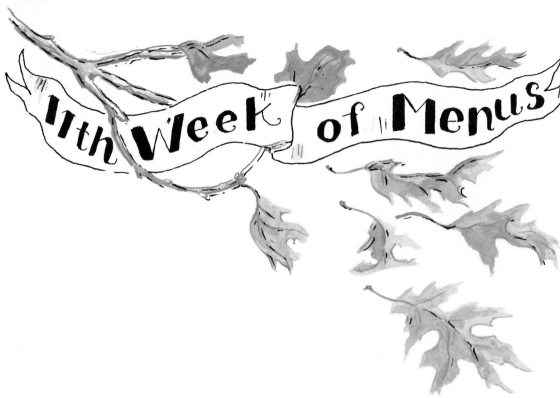

11th Week of Menus

Sunday

BREAKFAST

Orange Slices
*Breakfast Custard Pudding
Bacon

LUNCH

*Tuna-Celery Mold
Roll with Butter
Green Pepper and Carrot Sticks
Apple
Skim Milk

DINNER

Beef Roast
Potato with Butter
*Cauliflower Salad
Fruit Cup
Skim Milk

Monday

BREAKFAST

Apple Juice
Scrambled Egg
sprinkled with Parmesan Cheese
Toast with Butter
Whole Milk

LUNCH

*Shrimp Salad
*Working Woman's Bran Muffins
Broccoli
Tomato Wedge
Melon Balls
Skim Milk

DINNER

*Polynesian Chicken Livers
Buttered Rice
Broccoli
Whole Milk

Tuesday

BREAKFAST

Orange Juice
Peanut Butter
on English Muffin Half
Skim Milk

LUNCH

Chicken Breast
Italian Bread
*Ratatouille
Apple Slices
Skim Milk

DINNER

*Pork Chops with Red Cabbage
Green Beans
Parsleyed Potato with Butter
Applesauce
Whole Milk

Wednesday

BREAKFAST

Grapefruit Half
Poached Egg on Toast
Whole Milk

LUNCH

*Spinach Quiche
Whole Wheat Roll
Asparagus
Apple
Skim Milk

DINNER

*Fish Roll-Ups
*Parsley-Carrots-Potatoes
Green Beans
*Frozen Pineapple Dessert

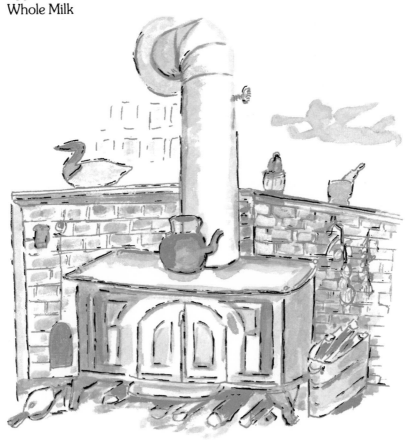

Thursday

BREAKFAST

Orange Juice
*Baked French Toast
Whole Milk

LUNCH

*Souffle Tuna Aspic on
Shredded Lettuce
Whole Wheat Roll with Butter
Tomato Slices
Apple
Skim Milk

DINNER

*Venison Roast
Buttered Noodles
*Vegetable Goulash
Fruit Salad
Skim Milk

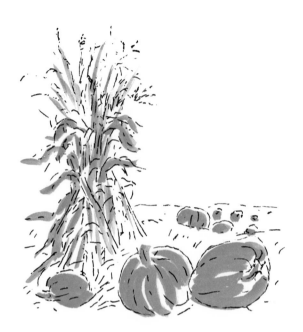

Friday

BREAKFAST

Pineapple Juice
Broiled Cheese on English Muffin Half
Whole Milk

LUNCH

Sliced Venison on Kimmelwick Roll
*Life Saver Soup
Orange
Skim Milk

DINNER

*Slim Jim Baked Chicken
Boiled Potatoes with Butter and Chives
French Beans
Carrots
Strawberry/Banana Slices
Milk

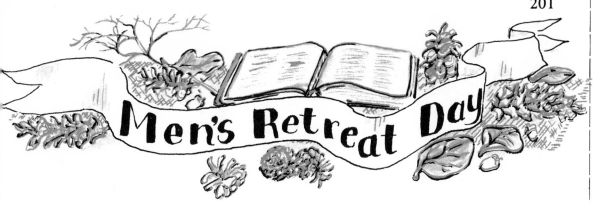

Men's Retreat Day

Friday

BREAKFAST

Grapefruit Half
Slice Fully Cooked Ham
*Baked French Toast
Whole Milk

LUNCH

Tacos (3 each) with Ground Beef Filling,
Tomato, Lettuce, Onion and Cheese
Buttered Carrots
*Peach Pie

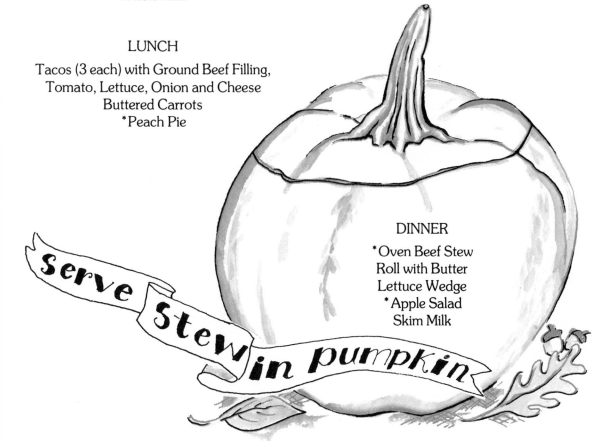

DINNER

*Oven Beef Stew
Roll with Butter
Lettuce Wedge
*Apple Salad
Skim Milk

serve stew in pumpkin

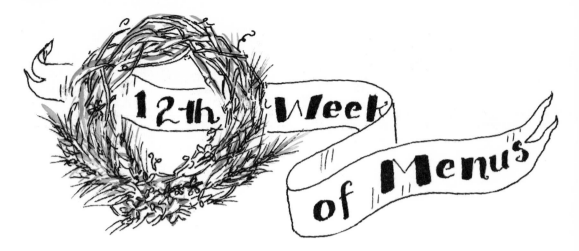

12th Week of Menus

Sunday	Monday
BREAKFAST	**BREAKFAST**
Broiled Grapefruit Half	Tangerine
Scrambled Egg	Cheese
*Johnny Cake with Butter	Cereal
Whole Milk	Whole Milk
LUNCH	**LUNCH**
*Salmon Croquettes	Open-Faced Sandwich
*Rye Roll with Butter	*Cabbage Soup
French-style Green Beans	Cucumber Strips
Relish Tray	Mandarin Orange
Apple	Skim Milk
Skim Milk	
	DINNER
DINNER	*Broiled Scallops
*Pot Roast Supreme	*Baked Tomato and Onions
Potato with Butter	*Carrot-Raisin Salad
Carrots	Whole Milk
Brussels Sprouts	
*Strawberry Julies	

Wednesday

BREAKFAST

Lowfat Cottage Cheese
Cereal with Skim Milk

Tuesday

BREAKFAST

Apple Juice
*Broiled Cottage Cheese on Toast
Bacon
Whole Milk

LUNCH

*Eggs Delmonico
Carrot Sticks
French Style Green Beans
Peach
Skim Milk

LUNCH

*Vegetable Cheese Soup
Julienne Salad with Leftover Meat
Leftover Vegetables
Lettuce with Low-Calorie Dressing
Crackers
Orange

DINNER

*Meatball Soup
Romaine Salad
Low-Calorie Dressing
*Ginger Fruit Cocktail
Skim Milk

DINNER

*Pork Belgian with Kraut
*Potato Bread with Butter
*Green Salad Vinaigrette
Applesauce
Skim Milk

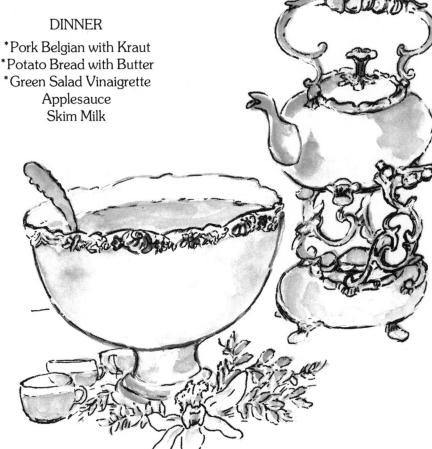

BREAKFAST

Sectioned Orange
Scrambled Egg
*Working Woman's Bran Muffin
Skim Milk

LUNCH

*Swiss Cheese Hawaiian
Whole Wheat Roll
Skim Milk

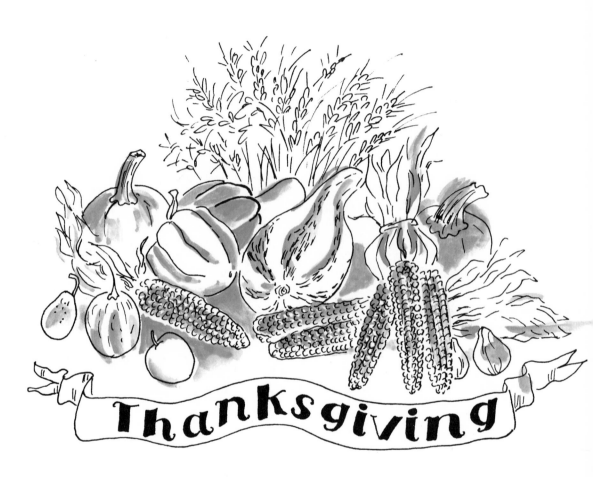

Thanksgiving

DINNER

*Mushroom Cocktail
Roast Turkey with
*Cornbread Stuffing
Mashed Potatoes
*Cranberry Chutney
*French Almond Green Beans
*Marinated Vegetable Medley
*Apple Compote

Friday

BREAKFAST

*Breakfast Cobbler
Bacon

LUNCH

*Seafood Salad Plate
*Potato Bread
Lettuce
Tomato Slices
Pear
Skim Milk

DINNER

*Veal Marengo
Brussels Sprouts
Raw Vegetable Platter
*Baked Peach Half
Whole Milk

Saturday

BREAKFAST

Raisins
Egg Over Easy
*Bran Muffin
Skim Milk

LUNCH

Hot Dogs
Baked Beans
Celery — Pickles
Cauliflower
*Berry Shake

DINNER

*Pork Stir-fry
Rice
Chinese Vegetables
*Unsweetened Applesauce
Skim Milk

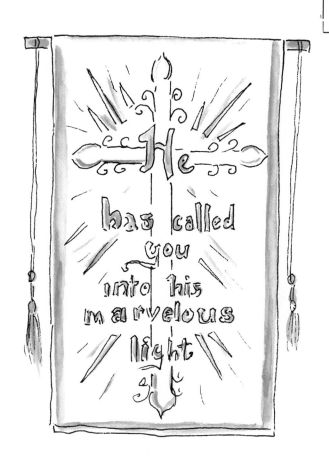

He has called you into his marvelous light

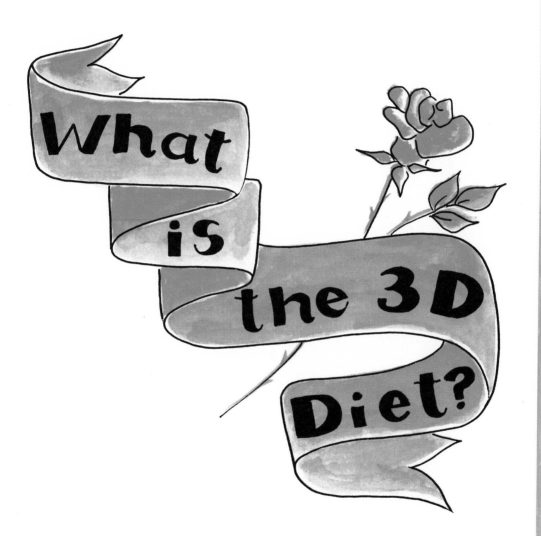

What is the 3D Diet?

What Is the 3D Diet?

The diet that 3D uses is based on the *Food Exchange List for Meal Planning*, developed by the American Dietetic Association and the American Diabetes Association, in conjunction with the National Institute for Health. These lists enable an individual to control his or her caloric intake, while enjoying meals with the rest of the family. In other words, you don't have to be on a "special diet." You can have what the others are having — up to a point; while they might be enjoying occasional ice cream or pie, you would be having a fruit exchange (one of the many foods listed in the fruit group).

The exchange lists divide our basic food requirements into six food groups: milk, vegetables, fruit, bread (which includes things like potatoes, peas, corn, and cereals), meat, and fat. The foods are listed in these categories according to similar vitamin, mineral, carbohydrate, and fat content, so that each group provides its own particular type of nutrients. Thus, given one bread exchange (which contains 15 grams of carbohydrates, 2 grams of protein, and 70 calories), for one piece of white bread we may substitute ("exchange") half a cup of bran flakes, a small potato, or even three cups of popcorn.

The important thing is to substitute *within* each group, and not from group to group. (You can't substitute a meat exchange for a milk exchange, for instance.) What makes this diet so effective is that it teaches the need for *balance* in eating. We learn to maintain the right balance of meat, bread, fruit, vegetables, milk, and fats, depending on the number of calories we should be consuming each day. This balance reflects the latest thinking in the field of nutrition, and it is the main reason why so many people consider it the soundest, most practical, common-sense diet they have ever tried, and why it really does re-pattern one's eating habits. It is also the most unboring diet. Even given the relatively few exchanges available on the 1000-calorie-a-day diet, it is still possible to use imagination and plan appetizing meals, including "gourmet-style" foods, as can be seen in the menu-planning section of this book.

A word about quantities: it is important to weigh and measure your food according to the amounts listed, as we are very much deceived by our own eyes. (It is an amazing thing to measure a 2-inch apple and see how small it is!) This self-deception is especially noticeable in the fat exchange list. By habit, we use much more butter or margarine than we realize — and need — yet one teaspoon to spread on toast is not very much! On the other hand, that teaspoon contains exactly twice as many calories as a teaspoon of sugar.

For those of you who are already familiar with the exchange lists, the fat exchanges have been revised to show the differences in the kind of fat — saturated and polyunsaturated. The former has now been definitely associated with an increase in blood cholesterol (a possible risk factor in coronary heart disease), while the latter has been associated with a *decrease* in blood cholesterol. Your physician may well advise you to substitute polyunsaturated fats for saturated fats wherever possible, and therefore low-fat foods, or those high in polyunsaturated fats have been set in **boldface** for your convenience.

appendix

The meat group will also represent a change. As stated above, fat has many calories that are present in meat, and they are one of the reasons for greater clarification in the meat group — to low, medium, and high-fat meats. A frankfurter, for instance, equals one fat exchange, as well as one meat exchange. As you can see, it would be easy to actually gain weight by eating too much of the high-fat meats.

Good luck on your diet! The Food Exchange List may not be new, but your approach to dieting takes on a new slant when you ask Jesus to help you "exchange" your old eating habits for His new ones!

Loretta Jack, Registered Dietitian

List 1*

Milk Exchanges

One Milk Exchange contains 12 grams of carbohydrate, 8 grams of protein, a trace of fat and 90 calories.**

Concerning a Milk Exchange, those which appear below in **bold type** are **non-fat.** Low-fat and whole milk contain saturated fat.

Non-fat Fortified Milk
Skim or non-fat	1 cup
Powdered (non-fat dry, before adding liquid)	⅓ cup
Canned evaporated skim milk	½ cup
Buttermilk made from skim milk	1 cup
Yogurt made from skim milk (plain, unflavored)	1 cup

Low-fat Fortified Milk
1% fat fortified milk (omit ½ Fat Exchange)	1 cup
2% fat fortified milk (omit 1 Fat Exchange)	1 cup
Yogurt made from 2% fortified milk (plain, unflavored) (omit 1 Fat Exchange)	1 cup

Whole Milk (omit 2 Fat Exchanges)
Whole milk	1 cup
Canned evaporated whole milk	½ cup
Buttermilk made from whole milk	1 cup
Yogurt made from whole milk (plain, unflavored)	1 cup

*The exchange lists are based on material in the *Exchange Lists for Meal Planning* prepared by Committees of the American Diabetes Association, Inc. and the American Dietetic Association, in cooperation with the National Institute of Arthritis, Metabolism and Digestive Diseases and the National Heart and Lung Institute, National Institutes of Health, Public Health Service, U. S. Department of Health, Education and Welfare.

**The calories vary depending on what kind of milk you choose. One exchange of skim-lowfat is 90 calories; low-fat is 120 calories; whole is 150 calories.

List 2
Vegetable Exchanges

One Vegetable Exchange contains about 5 grams of carbohydrate, 2 grams of protein and 25 calories. One exchange equals one-half cup.

Artichoke-½ medium	Leeks
Asparagus	Mushrooms, cooked
Bean sprouts	Okra
Beets	Onions
Broccoli	Pea Pods
Brussel Sprouts	Peppers
Cabbage, cooked	Rhubarb
Carrots	Rutabaga
Cauliflower	Sauerkraut
Collards	String Beans
Eggplant	green, wax, Italian
Green Pepper	Summer Squash (crooked neck)
Greens:	Tomato (1 large)
Beet	Tomato/Vegetable juice
Chards	Turnips
Dandelion	Water Chestnuts
Kale	Zucchini
Mustard	
Spinach	
Turnip	

The following raw vegetables may be used as desired:

Celery	Hot Peppers
Chicory	Lettuce
Cabbage	Mushrooms
Chinese Cabbage	Parsley
Cucumbers	Radishes
Endive	Spinach
Escarole	Watercress
Green onions	Zucchini

Starchy vegetables will be found in the Bread Exchange List.

appendix

List 3
Fruit Exchanges

One Fruit Exchange contains 10 grams of carbohydrate and 40 calories. Kinds and amounts of fruits to use for one Fruit Exchange:

Apple	2″	Mandarin oranges	¾ cup
Apple juice	½ cup	Mango	½ small
Applesauce	½ cup	Melon	
(unsweetened)		Canteloupe	⅓ 5″
Apricots, fresh	4	Honeydew	⅛ medium
canned	½ cup or 4 halves	cubes	1 cup
Banana	9″ long	Watermelon cubes	1¼ cup
Berries		Nectarine	1½″
Blackberries	¾ cup	Orange	2½″
Blueberries	¾ cup	Orange juice	½ cup
Raspberries	1 cup	Papaya	1 cup
Strawberries	1¼ cup	Peach	2¾″ or ¾ cup
Cherries	12 large	Pear	½ large or 1 small
canned	½ cup	Persimmon, native	2 medium
Cider	⅓ cup	Pineapple, raw	¾ cup
Cranberry Juice	⅓ cup	Dried fruit	¼ cup
canned	⅓ cup	Pineapple juice	½ cup
Dates	2	Plums (2)	2″
Figs, fresh (2)	2″	Prunes	3 medium
Fruit cocktail, canned	½ cup	Prune juice	⅓ cup
Grapefruit	½ medium	Tangerine (2)	2½″
Grapefruit segments	¾ cup		
Grapes	15 small		
Grape juice	⅓ cup		

Dried

Apples	4 rings	Figs	1½
Apricots	7 halves	Prunes	3 medium
Dates	2½ medium	Raisins	2 Tbsp

List 4
Bread Exchanges
(including bread, cereal, and starchy vegetables)

One Bread Exchange contains 15 grams of carbohydrate, 2 grams of protein, and 70 calories.

Bread

White (including French and Italian)	1 slice
Whole wheat	1 slice
Rye or pumpernickel	1 slice
Raisin (unfrosted)	1 slice
Bagel, small	½
English muffin, small	½
Plain roll, bread	1 (1 oz.)
Frankfurter roll	½
Hamburger bun	½
Dried bread crumbs	3 tablespoons
Tortilla, 6-inch	½ 6″

Cereal

Bran cereal, concentrated	⅓ cup
Bran flakes	½ cup
(All Bran, Bran Buds)	
Other ready-to-eat unsweetened cereal	¾ cup
Puffed cereal (unfrosted)	1½ cups
Cereal (cooked)	½ cup
Grapenuts	3 tablespoons
Grits (cooked)	½ cup
Rice, white or brown	⅓ cup
Pasta (cooked) spaghetti, noodles, macaroni	½ cup
Popcorn (popped, no fat added, large kernel)	3 cups
Cornmeal (dry)	2½ tablespoons
Flour	2½ tablespoons
Wheat germ	3 tablespoons
Shredded Wheat	½ cup

Crackers

Animal	8
Arrowroot	3
Graham, 2½ inch squares	3
Matzoth, 4 × 6	¾ oz.
Oyster	24
Pretzels, 3″ long × ⅛″ diameter	25 or ¾ oz.
Rye wafers, 2 × 3½	4
Saltines	6
Soda, 2½″ square	4
Whole wheat crackers (Finn, Kaoli, Wasa)	2-4 slices, ¾ oz.

Dried Beans, Peas, Lentils

Beans, peas, lentils (dried and cooked)	⅓ cup
Baked beans, no pork (canned)	¼ cup

Starchy Vegetables

Corn	½ cup
Corn on the cob	1 small, 6″ long
Lima beans	½ cup
Parsnips	⅔ cup
Peas, green	½ cup
Potato, baked	1 small, 3 oz.
Potato, mashed	½ cup
Winter squash, acorn or butternut	¾ cup
Yam or sweet potato	⅓ cup

Prepared Foods—Omit 1 fat also

Biscuit, 2½″ diameter	1
Chow mein noodles	½ cup
Cornbread, 2 × 2 × 1	1 2 oz.
Crackers, round butter type	5
Muffin, plain small	1
Potatoes, French fried, length 2-3½″	10
Pancake, 4 × ½″	2
Waffle, 4 × ½″	1
Stuffing	¼ cup
Taco shell	2, 6″
Whole wheat crackers	4-6

appendix

List 5
Meat Exchanges

One **Lean Meat Exchange** (1 ounce) contains 7 grams of protein, 3 grams of fat, and 55 calories.

Kinds and amounts of lean meat and other protein-rich foods to use for one Low-fat Meat Exchange are as follows. Trim off all visible fat.

Beef:	USDA Good or Choice grades of lean beef, such as round, sirloin, and flank steak; tenderloin; and chipped beef.	1 oz.
Pork:	Lean pork, such as fresh ham; canned, cured or boiled ham; Canadian bacon, tenderloin.	1 oz.
Veal:	All cuts are lean except for veal cutlets (ground or cubed). Examples of lean veal are chops and roasts.	1 oz.
Poultry:	Chicken, turkey, Cornish hen (without skin)	1 oz.
Fish:	All fresh and frozen	1 oz.
	Crab, lobster, scallops, shrimp, clams (fresh or canned in water)	2 oz.
	Oysters	6 medium
	Tuna (canned in water)	¼ cup
	Herring (uncreamed or smoked)	1 oz.
	Sardines (canned)	2 medium
Wild Game:	Venison, rabbit, squirrel	1 oz.
	Pheasant, duck, goose (without skin)	1 oz.
Cheese:	Any cottage cheese	¼ cup
	Grated parmesan	2 Tbsp.
	Diet cheese (with less than 55 calories per ounce)	1 oz.
Other:	95% fat-free luncheon meat	1 oz.
	Egg whites	3 whites
	Egg substitutes with less than 55 calories per ¼ cup	¼ cup

One **Medium-fat Meat Exchange** (1 ounce) contains 7 grams of protein, 5 grams of fat, and 75 calories.

When using meats from this list, 1 exchange = 1 Meat Exchange + ½ Fat Exchange. For example: 2 eggs = 2 Meat Exchanges + 1 Fat Exchange.

This list shows the kinds and amounts of medium-fat meat and other protein-rich foods to use for one Medium-fat Meat Exchange. Trim off all visible fat.

Beef:	Most beef products fall into this category. Examples are: all ground beef, roast (rib, chuck, rump), steak (cubed, Porterhouse, T-bone), and meatloaf	1 oz.

Pork:	Most pork products fall into this category. Examples are: chops, loin roast, Boston butt, cutlets.	1 oz.
Lamb:	Most lamb products fall into this category. Examples are: chops, leg, and roast.	1 oz.
Veal:	Cutlet (ground or cubed, unbreaded)	1 oz.
Poultry:	Chicken (with skin), domestic duck or goose (well-drained of fat), ground turkey	1 oz.
Fish:	Tuna (canned in oil and drained)	¼ cup
	Salmon (canned)	¼ cup
Cheese:	Skim or part-skim milk cheeses, such as:	
	Ricotta	¼ cup
	Mozzarella	1 oz.
	Diet cheeses (with 56-80 calories per ounce)	1 oz.
Other:	86% fat-free luncheon meat	1 oz.
	Egg (high in cholesterol, limit to 3 per week)	1
	Egg substitutes with 56-80 calories per ¼ cup	¼ cup
	Tofu (2½″ × 2¾″ × 1″)	4 oz.
	Liver, heart, kidney, sweetbreads (high in cholesterol)	1 oz.

One **High-fat Meat Exchange** (1 ounce) contains 7 grams of protein, 8 grams of fat, and 100 calories.

When using meat from this list, 1 exchange = 1 Meat Exchange + 1 Fat Exchange. For example: 2 frankfurters = 2 Meat Exchanges + 2 Fat Exchanges.

This list shows the kinds and amounts of high-fat meat and other protein-rich foods to use for one High-fat Meat Exchange. Trim off all visible fat.

Beef:	Most USDA Prime cuts of beef, such as ribs, corned beef	1 oz.
Pork:	Spareribs, ground pork, pork sausage (patty or link)	1 oz.
Lamb:	Patties (ground lamb)	1 oz.
Fish:	Any fried fish product	1 oz.
Cheese:	All regular cheese, such as American, Blue, Cheddar, Monterey, Swiss	1 oz.
Other:	Luncheon meat, such as bologna, salami, pimento loaf	1 oz.
	Sausage, such as Polish, Italian	1 oz.
	Knockwurst, smoked	1 oz.
	Bratwurst	1 oz.
	Frankfurter (turkey or chicken)	1 frank (10/lb.)
	Peanut butter (contains unsaturated fat)	1 Tbsp.

appendix

List 6
Fat Exchanges

One Fat Exchange contains 5 grams of fat and 45 calories.

To plan a diet low in saturated fat, select only those exchanges which appear in **bold type.** These are polyunsaturated.

Margarine, soft (tub or stick)[1]	1 teaspoon
Diet margarine	1 tablespoon
Avocado (4″ in diameter)[2]	⅛
Oil (corn, cottonseed, safflower, soy, sunflower, olive[2], peanut[2])	1 teaspoon
Olives[2]	10 small or 5 large
Nuts and seeds:	
Almonds[2], cashews	1 tablespoon or 6 whole
Pecans[2]	2 large whole
Peanuts[2]	20 small or 10 large
Pumpkin seeds	2 teaspoons
Walnuts	2 whole
Nuts, other[2]	1 tablespoon
Mayonnaise[1]	1 teaspoon
Reduced calorie	1 tablespoon
Butter	1 teaspoon
Bacon fat	1 teaspoon
Bacon	1 crisp strip
Chitterlings	½ oz.
Coconut, shredded	2 tablespoon
Cream, light	2 tablespoons
Cream, sour	2 tablespoons
Cream, heavy	1 tablespoon
Cream cheese	1 tablespoon
Cremora	1 tablespoon
Lard	1 teaspoon
Margarine (regular stick)	1 teaspoon
Salad dressing (all flavors)	1 tablespoon
Reduced calorie	2 tablespoon
Mayonnaise type[1]	2 teaspoons
Reduced calorie	1 tablespoon
Salt pork	¼ oz.
Spray oil	free

[1]If made with corn, cottonseed, safflower, soy or sunflower oil, can be used on fat-modified diet.

[2]Fat content is primarily mono-unsaturated.

Index

index

index

index